# PAINFULLY RESILIENT

## A Comprehensive Guide to Coping with Chronic Pain

**CHARLENE GABE-BOWEN**

**ISBN:** 9798867137564

# Table of Contents

# Introduction

Living with chronic pain can be a daily struggle for those who experience it. Whether it's a result of an ongoing health condition or an injury that never fully healed, chronic pain can greatly impact a person's quality of life. While many may focus solely on the physical aspects of chronic pain, it's important to also address the emotional and mental toll it can take. In this chapter, we will explore the connection between chronic pain and emotional well-being, and discuss ways to find relief by tackling both physical and emotional pain points.

## Understanding Chronic Pain: Beyond the Physical

Living with chronic pain is more than just a physical experience. It affects every aspect of a person's life, including their emotional well-being. Understanding chronic pain beyond the physical symptoms is crucial to finding effective ways to manage it and improve one's quality of life.

When we think of chronic pain, we often focus on the tangible symptoms, such as muscle aches, joint stiffness, or persistent headaches. However, chronic pain goes far beyond these physical manifestations. It is a complex condition that can impact a person's emotions, mental health, and overall well-being.

One of the ways chronic pain affects our emotional state is through its ability to limit daily activities. When pain becomes a constant companion, it can restrict our ability to engage in activities we once enjoyed. This loss can lead to feelings of frustration, sadness, and even a sense of isolation. Additionally, the unpredictability and variability of chronic pain can cause anxiety and fear of flare-ups or worsening symptoms, leading to a constant state of heightened stress.

The emotional toll of chronic pain can also strain relationships. Family members and friends may struggle to understand the limitations imposed by the condition, leading to misunderstandings and conflict. Moreover, the constant focus on pain can lead to self-doubt, decreased self-esteem, and a loss of confidence.

It is essential to recognize the impact of chronic pain on emotional well-being because ignoring these aspects can hinder the healing process. By addressing both the physical and emotional pain points, individuals with chronic pain can develop a holistic approach to managing their condition.

Understanding chronic pain beyond the physical allows

individuals to explore various coping mechanisms, such as relaxation techniques, mindfulness, and stress management. By incorporating these practices into their daily routine, individuals can create a supportive environment that promotes emotional well-being.

## The Connection between Chronic Pain and Emotional Health

Living with chronic pain not only affects our physical well-being but also has a profound impact on our emotional health. The connection between chronic pain and emotional well-being is complex and interdependent. When we experience chronic pain, it's not uncommon to also struggle with emotions such as anxiety, depression, and stress.

One of the main reasons for this connection is the way chronic pain alters our brain chemistry. When we are in constant pain, our brains can become hypersensitive, leading to heightened emotional responses. This means that even minor stressors or negative emotions can feel amplified. The ongoing battle with pain can also lead to feelings of frustration, helplessness, and a sense of losing control over our bodies.

Moreover, the experience of chronic pain can disrupt our sleep patterns, making it difficult to get a good night's rest. Sleep deprivation, in turn, can worsen our emotional state, making us more susceptible to feelings of irritability, anxiety, and sadness. This vicious cycle of pain, sleep disruption, and emotional distress can be incredibly challenging to break.

Another factor that contributes to the connection between chronic pain and emotional health is the social impact of the condition. Living with chronic pain can be isolating, as it may limit our ability to engage in social activities and maintain relationships. This social isolation can lead to feelings of loneliness, sadness, and even contribute to symptoms of depression.

It's important to recognize and address the emotional aspects of chronic pain alongside the physical symptoms. By understanding the connection between chronic pain and emotional health, we can develop strategies to improve our overall well-being. Seeking support from healthcare professionals, therapists, or support groups can provide valuable resources and coping mechanisms. Additionally, practicing self-care activities such as meditation, relaxation techniques, and engaging in hobbies that bring joy can help alleviate some of the emotional burden.

Finding relief from chronic pain requires a holistic approach that addresses both the physical and emotional pain points. By acknowledging and addressing our emotional well-being, we can improve our ability to manage and cope with chronic pain, leading to a better quality of life.

## Mental Aspects of Chronic Pain: Anxiety, Depression, and Stress

Living with chronic pain can take a significant toll on our mental well-being. It's not uncommon for individuals with chronic pain to experience anxiety, depression, and high levels of stress. The constant battle with pain can feel overwhelming, leading to a wide range of mental health challenges.

Anxiety often goes hand in hand with chronic pain. The fear of experiencing a flare-up or worsening symptoms can create a constant state of worry. We may become hyper-vigilant, constantly on edge, and anticipating the next bout of pain. This heightened state of anxiety can interfere with our ability to relax, enjoy activities, and maintain healthy relationships.

Depression is another common mental health concern for individuals with chronic pain. The chronic nature of pain can leave us feeling hopeless and helpless. The limitations imposed by the condition can lead to a loss of interest in activities we once enjoyed, feelings of isolation, and a lack of motivation. These symptoms can contribute to a downward spiral, making it even more challenging to cope with the pain.

Stress is a constant companion for those living with chronic pain. The constant physical discomfort and the impact it has on daily life can create a significant amount of stress. This stress can manifest in physical symptoms such as headaches, muscle tension, and sleep disturbances. Additionally, the ongoing stress can further exacerbate pain, creating a vicious cycle.

Addressing the mental aspects of chronic pain is crucial for finding relief and improving our overall well-being. Seeking support from mental health professionals can provide valuable resources and strategies to cope with anxiety, depression, and stress. Therapies such as cognitive-behavioral therapy (CBT) can help us identify and challenge negative thought patterns, develop healthier coping mechanisms, and improve our overall mental well-being.

Incorporating stress management techniques into our daily routine can also help alleviate the mental burden of chronic pain. Activities such as deep breathing exercises, mindfulness meditation, and relaxation techniques can help calm our minds and promote a sense of peace and well-being. Engaging in activities that bring us joy, such as hobbies or spending time with loved ones, can also be beneficial for managing mental health challenges associated with chronic pain.

It's essential to remember that addressing the mental aspects of chronic pain is just as important as addressing the physical symptoms. By taking a holistic approach to managing chronic pain, we can improve our overall quality of life and find relief from the emotional toll it takes.

# 1 The Emotional Rollercoaster of Chronic Pain

Chronic pain is often described as a journey, a long and winding road with many twists and turns. But what many people fail to mention is the emotional rollercoaster that comes along with it. It's a ride that no one signs up for willingly, yet so many find themselves strapped in and unable to get off. The reality of living with chronic pain goes far beyond physical discomfort; it takes a toll on our mental and emotional well-being as well. In this chapter, we'll delve into the emotional aspects of chronic pain, from the initial struggles of getting a diagnosis to the ongoing challenges of managing and coping with it. So hold on tight, because this rollercoaster ride is far from over.

## Understanding Chronic Pain: Its Impact and Prevalence

Chronic pain is not just a physical ailment; it is a complex condition that affects every aspect of a person's life. Its impact goes far beyond the physical discomfort, seeping into emotional well-being, relationships, and overall quality of life. To truly comprehend the reality of chronic pain, we must explore its prevalence, its wide-ranging effects, and the implications it has on individuals and society as a whole.

According to the Institute of Medicine, chronic pain affects an estimated 100 million Americans, making it more prevalent than heart disease, cancer, and diabetes combined. It is a condition that knows no boundaries, affecting people of all ages, genders, and backgrounds. Whether it manifests as migraines, back pain, arthritis, or any other form, chronic pain disrupts the lives of those who experience it, often leaving them feeling isolated, misunderstood, and desperate for relief.

The impact of chronic pain is not limited to the physical realm. It takes a toll on mental health, with studies showing high rates of depression, anxiety, and even suicide among those living with chronic pain. The constant discomfort and limitations imposed by the condition can wear down an individual's resilience, leading to feelings of helplessness, frustration, and hopelessness. Additionally, the toll of chronic pain extends beyond the individual, affecting relationships with loved ones, work productivity, and overall societal well-being.

One of the most challenging aspects of chronic pain is its unpredictability. Pain levels can fluctuate from day to day, or even within the same day, making it difficult for individuals to plan and participate in activities they once enjoyed. The chronic pain journey is often marked by a series of losses – the loss of independence, the loss of a career, and the loss of identity. The constant adaptation required to manage the pain can be mentally exhausting and emotionally draining.

The financial burden of chronic pain is also significant. Healthcare costs, medications, and therapies can quickly accumulate, placing a heavy strain on individuals and their families. Moreover, the impact of chronic pain on employment can lead to financial instability, further exacerbating the stress and emotional toll of the condition.

Understanding the prevalence and impact of chronic pain is crucial for healthcare providers, policymakers, and society as a whole. It is not simply a matter of physical pain; it is a public health issue that demands attention, resources, and compassionate support. Without proper understanding and acknowledgment of chronic pain's impact, those affected may continue to face skepticism, stigma, and limited access to appropriate care.

As we strive to raise awareness and improve the management of chronic pain, it is essential to address the barriers that individuals face in obtaining an accurate diagnosis and appropriate treatment. The complex nature of chronic pain often leads to a lengthy and frustrating journey of seeking answers. Misdiagnosis, lack of understanding, and dismissive attitudes from healthcare professionals can leave individuals feeling invalidated and further delay their access to necessary interventions.

Chronic pain management requires a multidisciplinary approach, incorporating not only medical interventions but also psychological support, physical therapy, and self-care strategies. However, accessing these resources can be a challenge, particularly for those with limited financial means or inadequate insurance coverage. Creating a healthcare system that is more inclusive and holistic in its approach to chronic pain is crucial to ensure that everyone can receive the comprehensive care they deserve.

## Navigating the Diagnosis Process: Patience, Perseverance and Medical Encounters

One of the most frustrating and challenging aspects of living with chronic pain is the lengthy and often arduous journey to obtain an accurate diagnosis. Many individuals with chronic pain can attest to the countless doctor's appointments, medical tests, and consultations that are often met with confusion, dismissal, and misdiagnosis. It is a process that requires patience, perseverance, and a willingness to advocate for oneself.

Patience is key when navigating the diagnosis process. It can take months, or even years, to find a healthcare professional who truly understands chronic pain and is able to provide an accurate diagnosis. During this time, it is important to resist the urge to become disheartened or give up. Keep in mind that finding the right diagnosis is essential for developing an effective treatment plan and finding relief. Trust your instincts and don't settle for answers that don't feel right or align with your experiences.

Perseverance is another crucial trait to possess when seeking a diagnosis for chronic pain. The road to diagnosis is often filled with dead ends, setbacks, and frustrations. It may require visiting multiple specialists, undergoing numerous tests, and even seeking second or third opinions. It can be exhausting, both physically and emotionally, but remember that each step forward brings you closer to understanding and managing your pain.

Medical encounters play a significant role in the diagnosis process, and they can be both empowering and disheartening. While some healthcare professionals are knowledgeable and compassionate, others may lack the understanding or expertise necessary to accurately diagnose and treat chronic pain. It is important to advocate for yourself and be an active participant in your own healthcare. Come prepared with a list of symptoms, questions, and concerns. Be persistent in seeking answers and don't hesitate to seek out a second opinion if necessary.

During medical encounters, it is crucial to communicate effectively with your healthcare provider. Be honest and transparent about your pain and its impact on your life. Share any relevant medical history, including previous diagnoses or treatments you have tried. Describe the intensity, duration, and specific characteristics of your pain, as well as any activities or factors that may aggravate or alleviate it. The more information you provide, the better equipped your healthcare provider will be to understand your condition and make an accurate diagnosis.

While the diagnosis process can be frustrating and disheartening, it is important to remain hopeful and optimistic. Remember that chronic pain is a complex condition, and there may not always be a straightforward answer or a quick fix. However, each medical encounter and test result provides valuable information that can help guide your treatment and management plan. Embrace the process as an opportunity for learning and growth, and never underestimate the power of perseverance.

In addition to patience, perseverance, and medical encounters, it is also crucial to engage in self-care throughout the diagnosis process. Living with chronic pain is emotionally and physically draining, and it is important to prioritize your mental and physical well-being. This can involve activities such as engaging in regular exercise, practicing stress management techniques, seeking support from loved ones or support groups, and exploring complementary therapies such as acupuncture or massage.

Lastly, it is important to acknowledge that the diagnosis process is not a linear journey. There may be setbacks, uncertainties, and moments of frustration along the way. It is normal to feel a range of emotions, including anger, sadness, and fear. Allow yourself to grieve the life you once had before chronic pain and embrace the necessary adaptations and adjustments that come with living with this condition. Seek out a supportive community of individuals who can relate to your experiences and offer guidance and empathy.

## Riding the Emotional Rollercoaster: Stress, Grief and Adaptation

Living with chronic pain is an emotional rollercoaster that can leave you feeling stressed, and grieving for the life you once had. The constant discomfort and limitations imposed by chronic pain can take a toll on your mental and emotional well-being, affecting every aspect of your life. In this section, we will explore the emotional challenges that come with chronic pain, including stress, grief, and the process of adaptation.

Stress is a common companion for those living with chronic pain. The daily struggle with pain can lead to increased stress levels, as you constantly navigate through physical discomfort and limitations. The stress of managing chronic pain can be relentless, as pain levels fluctuate and you are faced with the constant need to adapt and adjust. This chronic stress can have a negative impact on your overall well-being, contributing to feelings of anxiety, depression, and frustration.

Grief is another emotional response often experienced by those living with chronic pain. The loss of your former self, the life you once had, can be a significant source of grief. Chronic pain can force you to give up activities you once enjoyed, impacting your social life, hobbies, and even your career. It can be difficult to come to terms with these losses and adjust to a new reality. Grieving for the life you once had is a natural part of the chronic pain journey, and it is important to allow yourself to process these emotions.

Adaptation is a crucial component of living with chronic pain. As you navigate through the ups and downs of your pain journey, you will find yourself constantly adapting and adjusting to the challenges that come your way. This process of adaptation can be emotionally taxing, as it requires a significant amount of resilience, patience, and acceptance. It can be a rollercoaster of emotions, as you face setbacks and uncertainties along the way. But through it all, you have the opportunity to grow and discover new strengths within yourself.

One of the most important aspects of riding the emotional rollercoaster of chronic pain is finding healthy coping mechanisms. It is essential to develop strategies to manage stress and grief effectively. This can involve engaging in stress-reducing activities such as meditation, deep breathing exercises, or yoga. Finding outlets for emotional release, such as journaling or talking to a trusted friend or therapist, can also be beneficial. Taking care of your mental and emotional well-being is just as important as managing your physical pain.

Support from loved ones can be invaluable on this emotional rollercoaster. Surrounding yourself with understanding and empathetic individuals who can offer a listening ear or a shoulder to lean on can make a significant difference in your journey. Joining support groups or online communities with others who are experiencing similar challenges can provide a sense of belonging and validation. Sharing your experiences and connecting with others who truly understand can provide a much-needed source of support and comfort.

In addition to finding healthy coping mechanisms and seeking support, it is important to practice self-compassion. Living with chronic pain can often lead to feelings of guilt or self-blame, as you may struggle to meet the expectations you had for yourself before the onset of pain. Remember that chronic pain is not your fault, and it is essential to treat yourself with kindness and understanding. Be patient with yourself as you navigate through the emotional challenges, and celebrate your accomplishments, no matter how small they may seem.

Lastly, it is crucial to acknowledge that the emotional rollercoaster of chronic pain is not a linear journey. You may experience highs and lows, setbacks and breakthroughs. It is normal to have good days and bad days, both physically and emotionally. Embrace the process, and give yourself permission to feel a range of emotions. Remember that it is okay to ask for help when you need it, and to prioritize your mental and emotional well-being.

As you continue on your chronic pain journey, be gentle with yourself and allow yourself to ride the emotional rollercoaster. Remember that you are not alone in this experience, and there are resources and support available to help you navigate the challenges. By finding healthy coping mechanisms, seeking support, practicing self-compassion, and embracing the process of adaptation, you can find moments of peace and joy amidst the turbulence of chronic pain.

# 2 Exploring the Mind-Body Connection

While traditional treatments such as medication and physical therapy can provide relief, they often fail to address the root causes of pain. This is where the mind-body connection comes into play - the idea that our mental and emotional states can have a powerful influence on our physical health. In this chapter, we will explore the concept of the mind-body connection and how it can offer a holistic approach to coping with chronic pain.

## The Power of the Mind: Understanding the Mind-Body Connection

Chronic pain is a complex and multifaceted condition that can have a profound impact on every aspect of a person's life. From physical limitations and reduced mobility to emotional distress and decreased quality of life, chronic pain is more than just a physical sensation. It is a lived experience that affects the mind and body in intricate ways.

The mind-body connection is a concept that has been recognized for centuries and has gained significant attention in recent years. It suggests that our mental and emotional states can have a powerful influence on our physical health. In other words, our thoughts, emotions, beliefs, and attitudes can directly impact our physical well-being and, conversely, our physical health can influence our mental and emotional states.

Understanding the mind-body connection is crucial for those coping with chronic pain because it provides a holistic approach to pain management. Traditional treatments such as medication and physical therapy often focus solely on the physical aspects of pain, neglecting the psychological and emotional factors that contribute to the overall experience of pain. By acknowledging and addressing the mind-body connection, individuals with chronic pain can access a wider range of tools and techniques to manage their condition.

Research has shown that there are several mechanisms through which the mind-body connection influences pain perception and management. One such mechanism is the role of stress and anxiety. When we experience stress or anxiety, our body releases stress hormones such as cortisol, which can exacerbate pain sensations and increase the overall perception of pain. By learning to manage stress and anxiety through various techniques like deep breathing, meditation, and relaxation exercises, individuals can effectively reduce their pain levels and improve their overall well-being.

Another way the mind-body connection impacts pain management is through the release of natural pain-relieving chemicals called endorphins. These endorphins are produced in the brain and act as natural painkillers, promoting feelings of relaxation and well-being. By engaging in activities that stimulate the release of endorphins, such as exercise, laughter, and engaging in hobbies or interests, individuals can enhance their pain management abilities and experience a greater sense of control over their pain.

Additionally, the mind-body connection can influence pain perception through the power of perception itself. Our beliefs, expectations, and attitudes about pain can shape our experience of it. For example, individuals who have negative beliefs and expectations about their pain may experience more intense and persistent pain compared to those with positive beliefs and expectations. By shifting our mindset and adopting more positive and empowering beliefs about our pain, we can effectively reduce its impact and regain control over our lives.

Understanding the mind-body connection also highlights the importance of self-care and self-compassion in pain management. Chronic pain can often lead to feelings of frustration, anger, and hopelessness, which can perpetuate a cycle of suffering. By practicing self-care activities such as relaxation techniques, engaging in pleasurable activities, and seeking social support, individuals can cultivate a sense of well-being and resilience in the face of chronic pain. Self-compassion, which involves treating oneself with kindness and understanding, is also crucial in managing pain. By acknowledging our pain, validating our experiences, and practicing self-compassion, we can reduce the emotional distress associated with chronic pain and foster a positive mindset towards pain management.

## Practical Ways to Utilize the Mind-Body Connection for Pain Management

Living with chronic pain can be incredibly challenging, but understanding and harnessing the power of the mind-body connection can offer a new perspective and a wide range of tools to manage and cope with pain. In this section, we will explore practical ways to utilize the mind-body connection for pain management.

1. Mindfulness and Meditation: Mindfulness and meditation practices have gained significant attention in recent years for their ability to reduce stress, anxiety, and pain. These practices involve focusing your attention on the present moment and cultivating a non-judgmental awareness of your thoughts, feelings, and bodily sensations. By practicing mindfulness and

meditation regularly, you can develop a greater sense of calm, improve your pain tolerance, and enhance your overall well-being.

One simple mindfulness practice you can try is the body scan meditation. Find a quiet and comfortable space, close your eyes, and bring your attention to your body from head to toe. Notice any areas of tension, discomfort, or pain, and allow your breath to flow naturally, bringing a sense of relaxation to those areas.

2. Breathing Techniques: Deep breathing exercises are an effective way to calm your mind and relax your body, reducing the perception of pain. One technique you can try is diaphragmatic breathing. Sit or lie down in a comfortable position and place one hand on your chest and the other on your abdomen. Take a slow, deep breath in through your nose, allowing your abdomen to rise as you fill your lungs with air. Exhale slowly through your mouth, noticing the sensation of releasing tension and stress. Practice this breathing technique regularly to experience its benefits in pain management.

3. Guided Imagery and Visualization: Guided imagery involves using your imagination to create positive and calming mental images. By visualizing soothing scenes or pleasant memories, you can shift your focus away from pain and promote relaxation. Find a quiet space,

close your eyes, and imagine yourself in a serene and peaceful environment. Notice the details of the scene, engage your senses, and allow yourself to fully immerse in the experience. Guided imagery can be particularly helpful during moments of intense pain or discomfort, providing a distraction and promoting a sense of calm.

4. Progressive Muscle Relaxation: Progressive muscle relaxation is a technique that involves systematically tensing and relaxing different muscle groups in your body to release tension and promote relaxation. Start by sitting or lying down in a comfortable position. Focus on one muscle group at a time, starting with your toes and working your way up to your head. Tense each muscle group for a few seconds and then release, noticing the contrast between tension and relaxation. By practicing progressive muscle relaxation regularly, you can increase your body awareness, reduce muscle tension, and alleviate pain.

5. Cognitive-Behavioral Therapy (CBT): CBT is a type of psychotherapy that focuses on changing negative thoughts and behaviors that contribute to pain and distress. It involves identifying and challenging unhelpful thought patterns, developing coping strategies, and gradually changing behaviors that perpetuate pain. CBT can be particularly beneficial for individuals with chronic pain, as it helps to shift their

mindset and develop effective pain management skills. Consider seeking the guidance of a trained therapist who specializes in CBT to explore this approach further.

6. Physical Activity and Exercise: Engaging in regular physical activity and exercise has been shown to reduce pain, improve physical function, and enhance mood. Exercise stimulates the release of endorphins, the body's natural painkillers, and promotes the production of neurochemicals that improve mood and overall well-being. Find activities that you enjoy and can do safely within your pain limitations. It could be walking, swimming, yoga, or any other low-impact exercises. Start slowly and gradually increase the intensity and duration of your activities as you build strength and endurance.

7. Social Support: Chronic pain can be isolating, and having a supportive network of family, friends, or a support group can make a significant difference in your pain management journey. Connecting with others who understand your experience can provide emotional support, empathy, and helpful coping strategies. Consider joining local or online support groups, reaching out to friends and family, or talking to a mental health professional who specializes in chronic pain.

Incorporating these practical ways to utilize the mind-body connection for pain management into your daily routine can help you regain a sense of control over your pain, reduce its impact on your life, and enhance your overall well-being. Remember that each person's experience with chronic pain is unique, so it may take time to find the techniques and strategies that work best for you. Stay open-minded, be patient with yourself, and approach your pain management journey with curiosity and self-compassion. You deserve to live a fulfilling life, beyond the limitations of pain.

## Exploring Techniques and Strategies to Enhance Mind-body Interactions

When it comes to chronic pain, understanding the mind-body connection opens up a whole new world of possibilities for pain management. By exploring different techniques and strategies, you can enhance the interactions between your mind and body, ultimately leading to a reduction in pain and an improvement in overall well-being.

One technique to enhance mind-body interactions is biofeedback. Biofeedback is a method that allows you to monitor and gain control over certain bodily functions that are typically outside of conscious awareness, such as heart rate, blood pressure, and muscle tension. Through the use of sensors and monitoring devices, you can receive real-time feedback on these bodily functions and learn to regulate them through various techniques, such as deep breathing, relaxation exercises, and visualization. By becoming more attuned to your body's signals and learning to regulate your physiological responses, you can reduce pain and promote a greater sense of well-being.

Another strategy to enhance mind-body interactions is through the practice of yoga. Yoga combines physical postures, breathing exercises, and meditation to promote relaxation, flexibility, and strength. It has been shown to be effective in reducing pain, improving physical function, and reducing stress and anxiety. The physical movements of yoga can help release tension and promote a greater sense of body awareness, while the breathwork and meditation techniques can calm the mind and promote relaxation. By incorporating yoga into your routine, you can enhance the mind-body connection and find relief from chronic pain.

Meditative movement practices, such as tai chi and qigong, are also effective in enhancing mind-body interactions and reducing pain. These practices involve slow, flowing movements that are synchronized with deep breathing and mindful awareness. They promote relaxation, balance, and improved energy flow throughout the body. By engaging in these practices regularly, you can improve your body awareness, reduce muscle tension, and experience a greater sense of calm and well-being.

Acupuncture is another technique that has been used for centuries to enhance mind-body interactions and alleviate pain. It involves the insertion of thin needles into specific points on the body to stimulate energy flow and restore balance. Acupuncture has been shown to be effective in reducing pain, improving physical function, and promoting relaxation. By targeting specific acupoints, acupuncture can activate the body's natural pain-relieving mechanisms and promote overall well-being.

Aromatherapy is another strategy to consider when exploring mind-body interactions for pain management. Certain scents, such as lavender and peppermint, have been shown to have analgesic and relaxation effects. By inhaling these scents or using essential oils, you can stimulate the olfactory system and promote relaxation and pain relief. Incorporating aromatherapy into your daily routine can be as simple as using a diffuser, applying essential oils to your skin, or taking a soothing bath with scented bath salts.

Music therapy is another technique that can enhance mind-body interactions and reduce pain. Music has the power to evoke emotions, create a sense of calm, and distract from pain. Listening to calming and soothing music can trigger the release of endorphins, reduce stress hormones, and promote relaxation. Experiment with different genres and styles of music to find what resonates with you and provides the most pain relief.

Another strategy to enhance mind-body interactions is through the use of self-hypnosis. Self-hypnosis involves inducing a relaxed state and then utilizing suggestions or imagery to promote pain relief and relaxation. It can be a powerful tool for managing chronic pain by accessing the subconscious mind and reprogramming negative thought patterns and beliefs about pain. There are various resources available, including guided self-hypnosis recordings, books, and workshops, to help you learn and practice self-hypnosis techniques.

Finally, incorporating mindfulness practices into your daily life can greatly enhance the mind-body connection and promote pain relief. Mindfulness involves paying attention to the present moment without judgment and with an attitude of curiosity and acceptance. By bringing awareness to your thoughts, emotions, and bodily sensations, you can develop a greater sense of control over your pain and reduce its impact on your life. Mindfulness can be practiced formally through meditation, but it can also be integrated into daily activities, such as eating, walking, or engaging in hobbies. By cultivating a mindful approach to life, you can enhance the mind-body connection and find relief from chronic pain.

Exploring techniques and strategies to enhance mind-body interactions is a journey that is unique to each individual. It may involve trying different approaches, seeking guidance from professionals, and being open to new possibilities. By incorporating these practices into your daily routine, you can cultivate a greater sense of control over your pain, reduce its impact on your life, and promote overall well-being. Remember to approach this journey with curiosity, patience, and self-compassion. You deserve to live a life that is not defined by pain but is instead enriched by a harmonious mind-body connection.

# 3 Rewiring Your Brain for Pain Management Through Mindfulness

Despite the numerous treatments available, many people still struggle to find relief. However, there is a growing body of research that suggests mindfulness can be a powerful tool in managing chronic pain. By rewiring the brain and changing our relationship with pain, we can learn to cope with it in a more effective and empowering way. In this chapter, we will explore how adopting a mindfulness practice can help us reframe our perception of pain and improve our overall quality of life.

## The Science Behind Mindfulness and Pain Management

Chronic pain is a complex phenomenon that can often leave individuals feeling hopeless and frustrated. The traditional approaches to pain management, such as medications and physical therapies, may provide temporary relief but often fail to address the underlying causes of pain. This is where mindfulness comes in.

Mindfulness is a practice that involves intentionally bringing one's attention to the present moment without judgment. It encourages individuals to observe their thoughts, emotions, and bodily sensations without getting caught up in them. While mindfulness is often associated with mental health and stress reduction, recent research has shown its potential in managing chronic pain.

The link between mindfulness and pain management lies in the brain's ability to adapt and change. The brain has a remarkable capacity for neuroplasticity, which means it can reorganize and rewire itself based on our experiences and behaviors. Chronic pain is not just a physical sensation; it also involves cognitive, emotional, and behavioral responses. By practicing mindfulness, individuals can modify their brain's response to pain, leading to a reduction in pain perception and an improvement in overall well-being.

One of the key findings in the science of mindfulness and pain management is the role of the prefrontal cortex. This area of the brain is responsible for cognitive functions such as attention, decision-making, and emotional regulation. Chronic pain can lead to an overactivation of the pain-processing regions in the brain, such as the insula and the anterior cingulate cortex, while simultaneously reducing the activity in the prefrontal cortex. This imbalance can contribute to the amplification of pain signals and the experience of suffering.

Mindfulness practice has been found to strengthen the prefrontal cortex, thus restoring the balance between the pain-processing regions and the cognitive control regions. This enables individuals to regulate their emotional responses to pain and focus their attention on more helpful aspects of their experience. Research has also shown that mindfulness can reduce activity in the amygdala, which is responsible for fear and stress responses. By calming the amygdala, individuals can experience less emotional reactivity to pain, leading to decreased suffering.

Furthermore, studies have demonstrated that mindfulness can modulate the release of neurotransmitters and hormones involved in pain perception. Mindfulness has been shown to increase the production of endorphins, the body's natural painkillers, and decrease the levels of cortisol, the stress hormone. This neurochemical modulation can have a significant impact on pain management, as it promotes a sense of well-being and relaxation.

Another fascinating aspect of the science behind mindfulness and pain management is its effect on neuroplasticity. Regular mindfulness practice has been found to promote structural changes in the brain, particularly in regions involved in pain processing, such as the somatosensory cortex and the thalamus. These changes include an increase in gray matter volume, the density of neuronal connections, and the thickness of the cortical tissue. By rewiring these brain regions, individuals can experience a reduction in pain intensity and an improvement in pain tolerance.

It's important to note that the benefits of mindfulness for pain management are not limited to the physical realm. Chronic pain often takes a toll on mental and emotional well-being, leading to conditions such as anxiety and depression. Mindfulness practice has been shown to alleviate these psychological symptoms by reducing rumination, increasing self-compassion, and improving overall emotional regulation. By cultivating a non-judgmental and accepting attitude towards pain, individuals can develop a healthier relationship with their pain and decrease the negative impact it has on their mental health.

## Techniques for Adopting Mindfulness in Daily Routine

Once you understand the science behind mindfulness and pain management, you may be eager to incorporate it into your daily routine. Luckily, there are various techniques that can help you adopt mindfulness and reap its benefits in managing chronic pain.

1. Start with short meditation sessions: Meditation is a

key component of mindfulness practice, and it can be particularly helpful in managing chronic pain. Begin by dedicating a few minutes each day to sit in a quiet and comfortable space. Close your eyes and focus on your breath, bringing your attention to the sensations of inhaling and exhaling. As thoughts arise, simply acknowledge them without judgment and gently guide your attention back to your breath. Starting with shorter sessions can make it more manageable, and you can gradually increase the duration as you become more comfortable.

2. Engage in body scan exercises: Body scans are a valuable technique in mindfulness practice, especially for those dealing with chronic pain. This practice involves systematically scanning your body from head to toe, paying attention to any sensations or areas of discomfort. As you bring awareness to each part of your body, aim to observe the sensations without judgment or resistance. This practice can help you develop a deeper understanding of your body's signals and promote a sense of relaxation and acceptance.

3. Cultivate mindfulness in daily activities: Mindfulness doesn't have to be confined to meditation sessions alone. You can bring mindfulness into your daily routine by simply paying attention to the present moment during routine activities. Whether you're brushing your teeth, washing the dishes, or walking in

nature, try to bring your full attention to the task at hand. Notice the sensory experiences, such as the taste of toothpaste or the feeling of water on your hands. Engaging in activities mindfully can help you stay grounded and reduce stress and pain.

4. Practice mindful breathing throughout the day: Your breath is a powerful anchor that can bring you back to the present moment whenever you feel overcome by pain. Take a few moments throughout the day to focus on your breath. Notice the sensation of air entering and leaving your nostrils or the rise and fall of your belly. By intentionally directing your attention to your breath, you can cultivate a sense of calm and detachment from the pain.

5. Incorporate guided mindfulness exercises: If you find it challenging to practice mindfulness on your own, guided exercises can be a helpful tool. There are various resources available, including apps, websites, and YouTube channels, that offer guided meditations and mindfulness exercises specifically designed for pain management. These guided sessions can provide structure and support as you navigate your mindfulness practice.

6. Seek professional guidance: If you're new to mindfulness or would like to deepen your practice, consider seeking guidance from a qualified mindfulness

instructor or therapist. They can provide personalized strategies and support to help you integrate mindfulness into your daily life. They can also help address any concerns or difficulties you may encounter along the way.

7. Practice self-compassion: Living with chronic pain can be challenging, and it's essential to be kind and gentle with yourself throughout your mindfulness journey. Treat yourself with compassion and understanding as you navigate your pain. It's normal to have moments of frustration or resistance, but try to approach these emotions with self-compassion rather than judgment. Remember that mindfulness is a practice, and progress takes time and patience.

Remember, adopting mindfulness for pain management is not a one-size-fits-all approach. Experiment with different techniques and find what works best for you. Be open to adjusting and adapting your practice as needed. With consistent effort and a willingness to explore, mindfulness can become a valuable tool in managing chronic pain and improving your overall well-being.

Incorporating mindfulness into your daily routine may not provide an immediate cure for your chronic pain, but it can significantly improve your quality of life. By rewiring your brain and changing your relationship with pain, you can find empowerment and relief in the face of chronic pain. So why not give it a try? Start small, be patient with yourself, and embrace the journey towards a more mindful and pain-free life.

## Real-Life Success Stories of People Using Mindfulness for Pain Management

Mindfulness has gained popularity as a powerful tool in managing chronic pain, and real-life success stories abound. These stories not only offer inspiration but also serve as a reminder that with dedication and practice, anyone can experience the transformative effects of mindfulness in their pain management journey.

One such success story comes from Jane, who had been struggling with chronic back pain for several years. Despite trying various treatments, including medications and physical therapy, she found little relief. Frustrated and tired, Jane decided to explore alternative approaches and stumbled upon mindfulness. Skeptical at first, she began incorporating short meditation sessions into her daily routine. Over time, Jane noticed a shift in her perception of pain. Instead of resisting and fighting against it, she learned to observe her sensations without judgment. With regular practice, Jane developed a greater sense of acceptance and found that her pain became more manageable. Mindfulness helped her cultivate a compassionate attitude towards herself and her pain, leading to increased overall well-being.

John's success story is another testament to the power of mindfulness in pain management. He had been living with fibromyalgia for many years, a condition characterized by widespread pain and fatigue. Like Jane, John had tried numerous treatments, but none provided long-term relief. Feeling frustrated and exhausted, he decided to give mindfulness a chance. With guidance from a mindfulness instructor, John learned to bring his attention to the present moment and accept his pain without judgment. Through body scan exercises, he developed a deeper awareness of his body's signals and became better equipped to manage his pain. With consistent practice, John found that his pain intensity decreased, and he regained a sense of control over his life. Mindfulness gave him the tools to live a more fulfilling and empowered life despite his chronic pain.

Susan's story illustrates how mindfulness can alleviate the emotional toll of chronic pain. She had been living with migraines for as long as she could remember, enduring frequent attacks that left her feeling helpless and anxious. Desperate for relief, Susan turned to mindfulness and discovered the profound impact it had on her emotional well-being. Through mindfulness meditation, she learned to observe her thoughts and emotions without getting caught up in them. This practice allowed her to develop a sense of detachment from her pain, reducing her emotional reactivity and decreasing the suffering that often accompanied her migraines. Susan found that mindfulness helped her cultivate a more positive outlook on life, enabling her to better manage her pain and regain a sense of joy and gratitude.

These real-life success stories demonstrate that mindfulness is not just a buzzword but a valuable tool in managing chronic pain. They highlight the transformative power of rewiring the brain and changing our relationship with pain. Mindfulness allows individuals to shift from a place of resistance and suffering to one of acceptance and empowerment.

However, it's important to note that mindfulness is not a quick fix or a cure-all for chronic pain. It requires dedication, patience, and consistent practice. Each person's pain journey is unique, and what works for one individual may not work for another. It's essential to approach mindfulness with an open mind and be willing to adapt the practice to suit your specific needs.

If you're considering incorporating mindfulness into your pain management routine, it's important to start small and gradually build up your practice. Remember that mindfulness is a skill that takes time to develop, so be patient with yourself and celebrate even the smallest victories along the way. Seeking guidance from a qualified mindfulness instructor or therapist can also be beneficial, as they can provide personalized strategies and support to help you navigate your pain journey.

Ultimately, the real-life success stories of people using mindfulness for pain management serve as a reminder that change is possible. By rewiring your brain and embracing a mindful approach, you can find relief, empowerment, and an improved quality of life. So, why not embark on your own mindfulness journey today? Start small, be consistent, and open yourself up to the transformative power of mindfulness. You deserve a life that is free from the constraints of chronic pain, and mindfulness can be the key to unlocking that freedom.

# 4 How to Develop Emotional Resilience in the Face of Chronic Pain

The constant physical discomfort, limitations in daily activities, and uncertainty about the future can take a toll on one's mental and emotional well-being. However, amidst the struggles, it is possible to develop emotional resilience and maintain a positive outlook on life. In this chapter, we will explore the concept of emotional resilience and provide practical tips on how to cultivate it in order to cope with chronic pain. By incorporating these strategies into your life, you can stay strong and find inner strength to overcome the challenges of living with chronic pain.

## What is Emotional Resilience and Why it Matters in Managing Chronic Pain

Living with chronic pain can be an immense challenge, both physically and emotionally. The constant discomfort and limitations can wear a person down, affecting their mental and emotional well-being. That's where emotional resilience comes in.

Emotional resilience is the ability to adapt and bounce back from difficult situations, including chronic pain. It involves being able to navigate through the pain and its impact on daily life while still maintaining a positive outlook. Emotional resilience doesn't mean that you ignore or minimize your pain; instead, it focuses on building inner strength and coping strategies to navigate through the challenges.

Developing emotional resilience is essential for managing chronic pain because it allows you to maintain a sense of control over your life, despite the pain. It helps you stay engaged in meaningful activities, maintain relationships, and take steps towards managing your pain effectively. Emotional resilience enables you to face the challenges head-on and find ways to adapt.

One key aspect of emotional resilience is understanding and accepting your pain. This involves acknowledging the impact it has on your life and embracing the reality of your situation. Acceptance does not mean giving up or resigning yourself to a life of suffering. Instead, it means recognizing that chronic pain is a part of your life, and focusing on finding ways to cope and thrive despite it.

Another important aspect of emotional resilience is self-care. Taking care of your physical and emotional well-being is crucial when dealing with chronic pain. This includes getting enough rest, eating well, engaging in activities that bring you joy, and seeking support from loved ones or professionals when needed. Prioritizing self-care helps build resilience by giving you the strength and energy to face the challenges of chronic pain.

Developing effective coping strategies is another vital component of emotional resilience. This involves finding healthy ways to manage stress, anxiety, and negative emotions that often accompany chronic pain. Techniques such as deep breathing exercises, meditation, journaling, or engaging in hobbies can help regulate your emotions and provide a sense of calm in the face of pain.

Building a strong support system is also essential for emotional resilience. Surrounding yourself with understanding and empathetic people who can offer emotional support can make a significant difference in managing chronic pain. Whether it's family, friends, or support groups, having a network of people who understand your struggles and provide a listening ear can provide the support needed to navigate through the challenges of chronic pain.

Finally, maintaining a positive mindset is crucial for emotional resilience. It's easy to become consumed by negativity and despair when living with chronic pain, but actively focusing on the positive aspects of life can help build resilience. This can involve practicing gratitude, finding joy in small moments, and challenging negative thoughts or beliefs about your pain.

## Techniques to Develop Emotional Resilience When Dealing with Chronic Pain

Living with chronic pain can be incredibly challenging, but developing emotional resilience can help you navigate through the difficulties and maintain a positive outlook on life. In this section, we will explore some practical techniques that can help you cultivate emotional resilience while dealing with chronic pain.

1. Mindfulness and Meditation: Mindfulness and meditation are powerful tools for managing chronic pain and building emotional resilience. By focusing your attention on the present moment, you can learn to accept and manage your pain without becoming overwhelmed by it. Regular mindfulness and meditation practices can help you develop a greater sense of calm and reduce the impact of pain on your emotional well-being.

2. Positive Affirmations: Positive affirmations are simple statements that you can repeat to yourself to counter negative thoughts and beliefs about your pain. By consciously replacing negative self-talk with

positive affirmations, you can shift your mindset and cultivate a more resilient outlook. For example, instead of saying, "I'll never be able to do the things I love because of my pain," you could repeat the affirmation, "I am capable of finding joy and fulfillment despite my pain."

3. Gratitude Practice: Cultivating a sense of gratitude can be particularly powerful when dealing with chronic pain. By focusing on the positive aspects of your life and expressing gratitude for them, you can shift your perspective and enhance your emotional resilience. Keeping a gratitude journal or simply taking a few minutes each day to reflect on what you're grateful for can help you find moments of joy and contentment, even in the face of pain.

4. Healthy Lifestyle Choices: Taking care of your physical and emotional well-being is essential for building emotional resilience. This includes getting enough sleep, eating a balanced diet, and engaging in regular physical activity within the limitations of your pain. By prioritizing your health, you can enhance your overall resilience and better cope with the challenges of chronic pain.

5. Seeking Support: Chronic pain can often make you feel isolated and alone. Seeking support from loved ones or joining a support group can provide a valuable

source of emotional support and understanding. Sharing your experiences with others who are going through similar challenges can help you feel less alone and provide you with valuable insights and coping strategies.

6. Engaging in Meaningful Activities: Despite the limitations of chronic pain, finding ways to engage in activities that bring you joy and fulfillment is essential for maintaining emotional resilience. Whether it's pursuing a hobby, volunteering, or finding creative outlets, participating in meaningful activities can help distract you from your pain and provide a sense of purpose and accomplishment.

7. Flexibility and Adaptability: Learning to be flexible and adaptable in the face of chronic pain is key to developing emotional resilience. This involves accepting that your pain may fluctuate and that you may need to make adjustments to your plans or routines. By embracing a mindset of adaptability, you can find alternative ways to engage in activities you enjoy and maintain a sense of control over your life.

Incorporating these techniques into your life can help you develop emotional resilience and maintain a positive outlook while dealing with chronic pain. Remember, it's okay to seek professional help if you need additional support in building emotional resilience. You are not alone, and with the right tools and mindset, you can navigate through the challenges of chronic pain and find inner strength.

## Acceptance and Commitment Therapy (ACT)

Acceptance and Commitment Therapy (ACT) is a therapeutic approach that can be particularly helpful for individuals living with chronic pain. This type of therapy focuses on acceptance, mindfulness, and committing to actions that align with one's values, even in the presence of pain. ACT aims to help individuals develop psychological flexibility and improve their quality of life, despite the challenges posed by chronic pain.

One of the fundamental principles of ACT is the acceptance of pain. Rather than trying to fight against or avoid pain, ACT encourages individuals to acknowledge and accept it as a part of their experience. This acceptance does not mean resigning oneself to a life of suffering or giving up on finding relief. Instead, it involves recognizing that pain is a part of the present moment and learning to be with it, without letting it control or define one's life.

ACT also emphasizes the importance of mindfulness in managing chronic pain. Mindfulness involves being fully present and engaged in the present moment, without judgment. By cultivating a mindful awareness of their pain, individuals can learn to observe their thoughts, emotions, and bodily sensations. This mindfulness practice allows for greater self-compassion and a shift in perspective, which can help individuals develop emotional resilience and cope with chronic pain more effectively.

Another key component of ACT is the identification of one's values and commitment to living a life that is in alignment with those values. Chronic pain can often disrupt one's ability to engage in activities that are important and meaningful. Through ACT, individuals can clarify what matters most to them and identify actions they can take, even in the presence of pain, to live a fulfilling life. This commitment to values provides a sense of purpose and motivation, despite the challenges posed by chronic pain.

ACT also encourages individuals to develop psychological flexibility, which involves the ability to adapt and respond effectively to the ever-changing circumstances of life. This flexibility is particularly important when living with chronic pain, as it allows individuals to adjust their behaviors and strategies in response to fluctuations in pain levels or limitations. By being open to new approaches and perspectives, individuals can find alternative ways to engage in activities that bring them joy and satisfaction.

In addition to acceptance, mindfulness, commitment to values, and psychological flexibility, ACT may also incorporate other techniques such as cognitive restructuring and behavioral activation. Cognitive restructuring involves challenging and modifying negative thoughts or beliefs about pain, while behavioral activation focuses on increasing engagement in positive and meaningful activities.

Acceptance and Commitment Therapy can be delivered in individual therapy sessions or in group settings. A trained therapist can guide individuals through various exercises and techniques to develop emotional resilience and enhance their quality of life. It is important to find a therapist who specializes in chronic pain and has experience in using ACT.

## Cognitive-Behavioral Therapy (CBT)

Cognitive-Behavioral Therapy (CBT) is another therapeutic approach that can be highly beneficial for individuals living with chronic pain. This type of therapy focuses on identifying and modifying negative thoughts, beliefs, and behaviors that contribute to emotional distress and worsen the experience of pain.

CBT recognizes the powerful connection between our

thoughts, emotions, and behaviors. It operates on the premise that our thoughts and beliefs can significantly impact our emotional and physical well-being. In the context of chronic pain, individuals may develop negative thought patterns such as catastrophizing (exaggerating the severity of the pain) or engaging in all-or-nothing thinking (believing that they must be completely pain-free to experience any enjoyment or fulfillment).

The goal of CBT is to help individuals identify and challenge these unhelpful thoughts and beliefs. By working with a therapist, individuals can learn to reframe their thinking, replacing negative thoughts with more balanced and realistic ones. This can help reduce the emotional distress associated with chronic pain and enhance emotional resilience.

CBT also emphasizes the importance of behavioral changes in managing chronic pain. It recognizes that our behaviors can reinforce or alleviate our pain experiences. For example, individuals may avoid activities that they believe will exacerbate their pain, leading to a cycle of physical deconditioning and further limitations. Through CBT, individuals can learn to gradually and systematically expose themselves to these activities, developing confidence and demonstrating to themselves that they can engage in meaningful activities despite their pain.

A key aspect of CBT is the use of relaxation techniques and coping strategies to manage pain-related distress. These techniques may include deep breathing exercises, progressive muscle relaxation, or guided imagery. By incorporating these techniques into their daily lives, individuals can experience a reduction in stress and anxiety, which can have a positive impact on their pain perception.

One of the unique strengths of CBT is its focus on teaching individuals practical skills that they can use independently. Through CBT, individuals can learn to become their own therapist, recognizing when negative thoughts or behaviors arise and employing the strategies and techniques they have learned to effectively manage them.

CBT is often delivered in individual therapy sessions, although group therapy formats are also available. The duration and intensity of CBT can vary depending on individual needs and preferences. Some individuals may find that a brief, structured intervention is sufficient, while others may benefit from longer-term therapy to fully integrate the skills and strategies into their lives.

It's important to note that CBT is most effective when it is tailored to the individual's unique experiences and needs. A trained therapist can work collaboratively with the individual to develop a personalized treatment plan that addresses their specific challenges and goals.

Incorporating CBT into your pain management journey can be highly empowering. By addressing the cognitive and behavioral factors that contribute to emotional distress and worsen the experience of pain, CBT can help individuals develop emotional resilience and enhance their overall well-being.

Remember, building emotional resilience takes time and practice. Be patient with yourself as you navigate the challenges of chronic pain and explore different strategies and therapies. With the right support and mindset, you can develop the tools and skills needed to thrive in spite of your pain.

# 5 The Power of Social Support and Relationships

While there are various methods of managing chronic pain, one often overlooked aspect is the power of social support and relationships. Having a strong network of friends, family, and loved ones can make a significant difference in how one copes with chronic pain. In this chapter, we will explore the importance of social support and relationships in managing chronic pain and how they can positively impact an individual's journey towards better pain management.

## The Role of Social Support in Coping with Chronic Pain

Chronic pain is not just a physical ailment; it also takes a toll on a person's mental and emotional well-being. The constant discomfort and limitations can lead to feelings of isolation, frustration, and despair. This is where the power of social support and relationships comes into play. Having a strong network of friends, family, and loved ones can make a significant difference in how one copes with chronic pain.

When faced with chronic pain, it's easy to become consumed by the physical aspect of the condition. But what many people overlook is the emotional toll it takes. It's not uncommon for individuals with chronic pain to feel depressed, anxious, or overwhelmed. This is where social support comes in. Having someone to talk to, to share your struggles with, can provide a sense of relief and validation. Knowing that there are people who understand and empathize with what you're going through can be incredibly comforting.

Social support also plays a crucial role in reducing the impact of stress on chronic pain. Stress has been known to exacerbate pain, making it more intense and difficult to manage. But having a support system in place can help alleviate stress. Simply talking to someone about your concerns and fears can provide a sense of relief and reduce stress levels. Additionally, engaging in activities with loved ones, whether it's going for a walk or watching a movie together, can serve as a distraction from the pain and help shift the focus to more positive experiences.

Furthermore, social support can empower individuals with chronic pain to take a more active role in their pain management. When you have people in your corner who believe in your ability to manage your pain, it can boost your confidence and motivation. It's much easier to tackle the challenges of chronic pain when you have a support system cheering you on and providing encouragement along the way.

One of the benefits of social support is the opportunity to learn from others who have faced similar challenges. Sharing experiences and strategies for managing pain can provide valuable insights and new perspectives. It can open doors to alternative treatment options or coping mechanisms that you may not have considered before. Hearing success stories from others who have found ways to improve their quality of life despite chronic pain can instill hope and inspire you to explore new possibilities.

In summary, social support and relationships play a vital role in coping with chronic pain. The emotional and practical support provided by friends, family, and loved ones can help alleviate the burden of pain and improve overall well-being. It's important to cultivate and nurture these relationships, as they can make a significant difference in managing chronic pain. Remember, you don't have to face chronic pain alone - reach out and lean on your support system for comfort, guidance, and strength.

## Strengthening Relationships to Manage Chronic Pain

Developing and strengthening relationships is essential for managing chronic pain. It is through these connections that individuals with chronic pain can find support, understanding, and encouragement. Here are some ways to strengthen relationships to better manage chronic pain:

1. Open communication: Effective communication is the foundation of any strong relationship. It is crucial to have open and honest conversations with your loved ones about your chronic pain and how it affects you. This will help them gain a deeper understanding of your condition and what you need from them in terms of support. It is important to express your emotions, fears, and concerns openly, as this can foster empathy and create a safe space for both you and your loved ones to share your thoughts and feelings.

2. Educate your loved ones: Chronic pain can be an invisible condition, making it difficult for others to fully comprehend its impact on your life. Take the time to educate your loved ones about your condition. Share information, resources, and personal experiences that can help them better understand what you are going through. This will enable them to provide more effective support and become better allies in your pain management journey.

3. Practice empathy and understanding: Strengthening relationships involves showing empathy and understanding towards one another. Your loved ones may not fully comprehend the extent of your pain, but

by practicing empathy, you can bridge the gap between their experiences and yours. Similarly, it is important to understand that your loved ones may not always know how to respond or help. Patience and understanding can go a long way in building strong relationships and managing chronic pain together.

4. Set realistic expectations: Chronic pain can sometimes limit your ability to engage in certain activities or attend social events. Setting realistic expectations with your loved ones can help alleviate feelings of guilt or frustration. Clearly communicate your limitations and find alternative ways to spend time together. This could involve engaging in activities that are less physically demanding, such as watching a movie or having a conversation over a cup of tea. By setting realistic expectations, you can maintain a sense of normalcy in your relationships while managing your pain effectively.

5. Seek professional support: Sometimes, it can be challenging for loved ones to fully comprehend the complexities of chronic pain. In these cases, seeking professional support can be beneficial. Couples counseling or family therapy can provide a safe space for open communication, address any misunderstandings or conflicts, and strengthen the support system around you. Professional guidance can help everyone involved navigate the challenges of

chronic pain more effectively.

6. Join support groups or communities: Connecting with others who are going through similar experiences can be incredibly empowering. Joining support groups or online communities focused on chronic pain can provide a sense of belonging, validation, and encouragement. These platforms offer a space to share experiences, exchange coping strategies, and receive support from individuals who truly understand what you are going through. These connections can not only strengthen your relationships but also help you discover new tools and techniques for managing chronic pain.

## Techniques to Leverage Social Support for Pain Management

Chronic pain can be a challenging journey, but with the power of social support and relationships, you can navigate it more effectively. Here are some techniques to leverage social support for pain management:

1. Communicate openly and honestly: Effective communication is key to leveraging social support. Express your needs, concerns, and emotions to your loved ones. Let them know how chronic pain affects you and what support you require. By sharing openly, you can create a safe space for both you and your loved

ones to understand and support each other.

2. Ask for help when needed: Don't hesitate to ask for help when you need it. It's okay to lean on your support system for assistance with daily tasks, appointments, or even just a listening ear. Remember that your loved ones want to help, and allowing them to do so strengthens your bond and relieves some of the burden.

3. Foster a positive support network: Surround yourself with individuals who are understanding, empathetic, and supportive. Seek out friends, family members, or support groups that can offer encouragement and guidance. Being a part of a positive support network can make a significant difference in your pain management journey.

4. Seek professional support: In addition to social support, it may be beneficial to seek professional help. A pain management specialist, therapist, or counselor can provide additional guidance and tools to help you navigate chronic pain. They can also support your loved ones in understanding your condition better.

5. Practice self-care: Taking care of yourself is essential in managing chronic pain. Engage in activities that bring you joy and help you relax. Set aside time for rest and prioritize activities that promote your physical and mental well-being. By caring for yourself, you'll have

more energy and resilience to lean on your support system effectively.

6. Attend support groups or therapy sessions together: If your loved ones are open to it, consider attending support groups or therapy sessions together. This can provide a deeper understanding of chronic pain and facilitate healthy discussions around how everyone can best support each other. Participating in these sessions as a team can strengthen your relationships and help you navigate pain management together.

7. Show gratitude and appreciation: Take the time to show gratitude and appreciation for the support you receive. A simple thank you can go a long way in acknowledging the efforts of your loved ones. Expressing gratitude fosters a positive and supportive environment, reinforcing the strength of your relationships.

8. Practice active listening: When engaging in conversations with your loved ones, practice active listening. Give them your full attention and validate their feelings and experiences. By truly listening, you show that their support is valued and appreciated. This strengthens the bond between you and enhances your support system.

9. Set boundaries and communicate your limitations:

Chronic pain may require you to set boundaries to protect your well-being. Communicate these boundaries to your loved ones and let them know your limitations. By setting clear expectations, you can avoid misunderstandings and maintain healthy relationships.

10. Celebrate milestones and achievements together: Whether it's a small victory or a significant milestone, celebrate your achievements together with your support system. Recognize and acknowledge the progress you've made in managing your pain. By celebrating together, you foster a positive environment and motivate each other to keep pushing forward.

Remember, you don't have to face chronic pain alone. Social support and relationships can be powerful tools in your pain management toolbox. Leverage these techniques to strengthen your relationships, foster understanding, and receive the support you need to thrive despite chronic pain. You have a network of individuals who care about your well-being and are ready to be there for you every step of the way. Embrace their support and let it empower you on your pain management journey.

## Personal Stories: Living With Chronic Pain Through Support

Living with chronic pain can be a lonely and isolating experience. It's easy to feel like no one truly understands what you're going through, and that can make the journey even more challenging. However, finding solace in personal stories from others who have lived through similar experiences can provide a glimmer of hope and a sense of belonging. In this section, we will share personal stories from individuals who have learned to navigate the ups and downs of chronic pain with the help of social support and relationships.

Emily has been living with chronic pain for over a decade due to a back injury. At first, she felt completely alone. It wasn't until she reached out to a support group for individuals with chronic pain that she found a sense of belonging. Through this group, she met others who shared their struggles, victories, and coping strategies. It was through these connections that Emily discovered new treatment options and techniques that helped alleviate her pain. She also found comfort in being able to openly share her experiences without fear of judgment or misunderstanding. Emily's support group became her lifeline, providing emotional support, understanding, and a safe space to navigate the challenges of chronic pain.

Mike was diagnosed with fibromyalgia several years ago, and it turned his life upside down. As his pain persisted, he found it increasingly difficult to maintain relationships and engage in activities he once enjoyed. However, with the support of his family and friends, Mike was able to regain a sense of normalcy. They took the time to educate themselves about fibromyalgia and understand the limitations it imposed on Mike's life. They adjusted their plans and activities to accommodate his needs, ensuring that he didn't feel left out or isolated. Mike's loved ones also provided a listening ear, offering him a space to vent his frustrations and fears. Their unwavering support helped him feel less alone and gave him the strength to persevere.

Sarah's chronic pain journey began after a car accident that left her with nerve damage in her legs. The pain was intense, and it took a toll on her mental health. She found herself withdrawing from her friends and family, convinced that they couldn't possibly understand her pain. It wasn't until she reached out to a therapist specializing in chronic pain that she learned the power of social support. With her therapist's guidance, Sarah began rebuilding her relationships, starting with small steps like inviting friends over for tea or going for short walks with family members. She discovered that her loved ones were more than willing to support her; they just needed her to let them in. Sarah's journey taught her the importance of vulnerability and how embracing her support system ultimately made her feel stronger and more empowered.

These personal stories highlight the transformative power of social support and relationships in the face of chronic pain. They demonstrate that no matter how isolated or overwhelmed you may feel, there are people out there who understand and are willing to walk alongside you on your journey. The connections formed through support groups, therapy, and open communication with loved ones can make a significant difference in managing chronic pain and improving overall well-being.

As you navigate your own chronic pain journey, remember that you are not alone. Reach out to support groups, seek therapy, and lean on your loved ones for support. Share your experiences, listen to the stories of others, and embrace the connections that can empower you to find new ways to manage your pain. Together, we can create a world where individuals with chronic pain feel seen, heard, and supported.

# 6 Self-Care for Chronic Pain: Tips to Live Your Best Life

While there may not be a cure for your pain, there are ways to manage it and improve your overall quality of life. One key aspect of coping with chronic pain is practicing self-care. By taking care of yourself physically, mentally, and emotionally, you can better manage your pain and live your best life. In this chapter, we'll discuss some essential lifestyle and self-care strategies that can help you cope with chronic pain and improve your well-being. From nutrition and sleep to exercise and stress management, we've got you covered with practical tips to help you live your best life despite chronic pain.

## The Correlation Between Nutrition and Chronic Pain

Living with chronic pain can significantly impact various aspects of your life, including your physical, emotional, and mental well-being. While there may not be a cure for chronic pain, managing it through self-care strategies can help improve your overall quality of life. One crucial aspect of self-care that often gets overlooked is nutrition. The correlation between nutrition and chronic pain is a topic that deserves attention, as the food we consume can play a significant role in managing and even reducing pain levels.

First and foremost, it's essential to maintain a well-balanced diet that is rich in nutrients. Certain foods have anti-inflammatory properties that can help alleviate chronic pain symptoms. Incorporating a variety of fruits and vegetables, whole grains, lean proteins, and healthy fats into your diet can help reduce inflammation and provide your body with the necessary nutrients for healing and overall well-being.

Omega-3 fatty acids, found in foods like fatty fish, flaxseeds, and walnuts, have been shown to have anti-inflammatory properties. Consuming foods high in omega-3s can help reduce pain levels and improve joint mobility in individuals with chronic pain conditions such as arthritis. Similarly, incorporating spices like turmeric, ginger, and garlic into your meals can provide natural pain-relieving benefits due to their anti-inflammatory properties.

In addition to consuming anti-inflammatory foods, it's crucial to avoid or limit foods that can increase inflammation in the body. Processed foods, refined sugars, trans fats, and excessive alcohol consumption have all been linked to increased inflammation and worsened chronic pain symptoms. By reducing or eliminating these foods from your diet, you can potentially reduce inflammation levels and manage pain more effectively.

Another important aspect of nutrition and chronic pain management is maintaining a healthy weight. Excess weight puts added strain on your joints and can worsen chronic pain symptoms. By focusing on a well-balanced diet and engaging in regular exercise, you can maintain a healthy weight and alleviate some of the stress on your joints, leading to reduced pain levels.

Hydration is also key in managing chronic pain. Dehydration can exacerbate pain and inflammation in the body, so it's crucial to drink an adequate amount of water throughout the day. Aim to consume at least eight glasses of water daily, and be mindful of your caffeine and alcohol intake, as these can contribute to dehydration.

Lastly, it's important to remember that everyone's body is unique, and what works for one person may not work for another. Keep a journal of your diet and note any patterns or correlations between certain foods and changes in pain levels. This will help you identify which foods may be triggering inflammation or exacerbating your chronic pain symptoms, allowing you to make more informed dietary choices.

## Mastering Sleep Strategies for Alleviating Chronic Pain

Getting enough quality sleep is crucial for everyone's overall well-being, but it is especially important for those living with chronic pain. Sleep is a time when our bodies heal and recharge, and lack of sleep can exacerbate pain levels and make it harder to cope with the challenges of daily life. However, with some practical strategies, you can master sleep strategies that alleviate chronic pain and improve your quality of life.

First and foremost, establishing a consistent sleep routine is essential. Try to go to bed and wake up at the same time every day, even on weekends. This helps regulate your body's internal clock and promotes better sleep quality. Create a relaxing bedtime routine that allows you to wind down and signal to your body that it's time for rest. This can include activities such as taking a warm bath, reading a book, or practicing relaxation techniques like deep breathing or meditation.

Creating a sleep-friendly environment is also crucial for getting a good night's rest. Ensure that your bedroom is dark, quiet, and at a comfortable temperature. Invest in a supportive mattress and pillows that align with your specific needs and provide proper spinal alignment. Consider using blackout curtains, earplugs, or a white noise machine to block out any external distractions that may disrupt your sleep.

Managing pain before bed is another important aspect of mastering sleep strategies for chronic pain relief. Develop a pre-sleep routine that includes pain management techniques, such as applying heat or cold therapy to affected areas, stretching or engaging in gentle exercises, or using over-the-counter pain relievers as recommended by your healthcare provider. By addressing pain before bed, you can increase your chances of falling asleep faster and experiencing less discomfort throughout the night.

Additionally, it's important to prioritize relaxation and stress reduction techniques before bedtime. Chronic pain often leads to increased stress and anxiety, which can interfere with sleep. Incorporate relaxation techniques into your evening routine, such as practicing mindfulness or deep breathing exercises, listening to calming music, or engaging in gentle yoga or stretching. Avoid stimulating activities or electronic devices that emit blue light, as this can interfere with your body's production of melatonin, the hormone responsible for regulating sleep.

Finally, if you're still struggling with sleep despite implementing these strategies, it may be beneficial to consult with a healthcare professional who specializes in sleep disorders. They can evaluate your specific situation and provide recommendations or prescribe medications if necessary to help improve sleep quality.

Remember, mastering sleep strategies for alleviating chronic pain is a trial-and-error process. It may take some time to find what works best for you, but don't give up. With patience and perseverance, you can establish healthy sleep habits that will not only improve your pain management but also enhance your overall well-being. Sleep is a powerful tool in your self-care arsenal, and by prioritizing it, you are taking a significant step towards living your best life despite chronic pain.

## The Role of Exercise in Chronic Pain Management

Regular exercise plays a vital role in managing chronic pain and improving overall well-being. It may seem counterintuitive to exercise when you're in pain, but physical activity has been shown to reduce pain levels and increase functionality in individuals with chronic pain conditions.

Engaging in regular exercise can help strengthen muscles, improve flexibility, and increase endurance, which can all contribute to better pain management. Exercise releases endorphins, the body's natural painkillers, which can help alleviate pain and improve mood. Additionally, exercise promotes better sleep, reduces stress, and increases overall energy levels, all of which can contribute to better pain management and quality of life.

When it comes to exercise and chronic pain, it's essential to find activities that work for you and your specific condition. Not all exercises are suitable for everyone, and certain movements or positions may aggravate your pain. Consult with your healthcare provider or a physical therapist to determine the best exercises for your condition and any modifications or adaptations that may be necessary.

Low-impact exercises, such as walking, swimming, cycling, or using an elliptical machine, are often recommended for individuals with chronic pain. These activities provide cardiovascular benefits without placing excessive stress on your joints. Water-based exercises, such as aqua aerobics or swimming, can be particularly beneficial as they provide buoyancy and reduce pressure on the joints.

Strength training exercises are also important for individuals with chronic pain. Building strength in your muscles can help support and protect your joints, reducing pain and improving functionality. Focus on exercises that target the specific muscles surrounding your problem areas, and start with light weights or resistance bands to avoid overexertion. Gradually increase the intensity as your strength improves.

Stretching and flexibility exercises can help improve range of motion and reduce muscle tension. Incorporate gentle stretching into your exercise routine, making sure to warm up your muscles beforehand to avoid injury. Yoga and Pilates can be particularly beneficial as they emphasize stretching, flexibility, and relaxation.

It's important to listen to your body and not push yourself too hard. Start slowly and gradually increase the duration and intensity of your workouts. If you experience increased pain or discomfort, modify your activities or take a break. Over time, as your body adapts to exercise, you may find that your pain levels decrease, and you can engage in more challenging workouts.

Remember, exercise should be enjoyable, not a chore. Find activities that you genuinely enjoy and that align with your interests and preferences. This will help increase motivation and make it easier to stick to your exercise routine. Consider joining a group exercise class, participating in a team sport, or finding an exercise buddy to help make your workouts more enjoyable and social.

Incorporating regular exercise into your self-care routine is an essential component of managing chronic pain. While it may be challenging at times, the benefits are well worth the effort. Consult with your healthcare provider, listen to your body, and find activities that work for you. With consistency and perseverance, you can harness the power of exercise to better manage your pain and live your best life.

## Effective Stress Management Techniques for Chronic Pain Relief

Living with chronic pain can be incredibly stressful. The constant discomfort, limitations on activities, and uncertainty about the future can take a toll on your mental and emotional well-being. That's why it's crucial to have effective stress management techniques in place to help you find relief and maintain a positive mindset.

One effective stress management technique for chronic pain relief is mindfulness meditation. Mindfulness involves focusing your attention on the present moment without judgment. This practice can help you become more aware of your pain without getting caught up in negative thoughts or emotions. By observing your pain from a place of detachment, you can reduce its impact on your mental state. Regular mindfulness meditation has been shown to decrease stress levels, improve mood, and increase pain tolerance.

Deep breathing exercises are another useful stress management technique for chronic pain relief. When you're in pain, your body tends to tense up, which can exacerbate your discomfort. Deep breathing helps you relax your muscles, release tension, and promote a sense of calm. Take slow, deep breaths in through your nose, hold for a few seconds, and then exhale slowly through your mouth. Focus on your breath and let go of any tension you may be holding in your body. Repeat this exercise several times a day.

Engaging in enjoyable activities can also help alleviate stress and manage chronic pain. Find hobbies or activities that bring you joy and make you feel good. Whether it's painting, playing an instrument, gardening, or dancing, doing something you love can take your mind off your pain and help you relax. These activities provide a sense of accomplishment and fulfillment, which can boost your mood and reduce stress levels.

Social support is crucial when it comes to managing stress and chronic pain. Reach out to friends, family members, or support groups who understand what you're going through. Having a support system can provide a safe space to express your feelings, receive empathy, and gain valuable advice. It's essential to surround yourself with people who are understanding and supportive of your situation.

In addition to these stress management techniques, it's important to establish healthy coping mechanisms. Avoid turning to unhealthy habits such as smoking, excessive alcohol consumption, or overeating as a way to cope with stress. Instead, focus on healthy coping mechanisms like exercise, journaling, listening to music, or practicing relaxation techniques. Find what works best for you and make it a regular part of your self-care routine.

Remember, managing stress is an ongoing process, and what works for one person may not work for another. Be patient with yourself as you explore different stress management techniques and find what resonates with you. It may take time and experimentation, but with perseverance, you can develop effective strategies to manage stress and alleviate chronic pain.

## Building Your Personalized Self-Care Plan for Chronic Pain

Living with chronic pain requires a personalized self-care plan that addresses your specific needs and challenges. While there are general strategies that can help manage chronic pain, it's important to tailor your approach to what works best for you. Building your personalized self-care plan involves understanding your pain triggers, identifying coping mechanisms, and incorporating activities that promote physical, mental, and emotional well-being.

Start by identifying your pain triggers and patterns. Keep a journal to track your pain levels throughout the day and note any activities, foods, or situations that may exacerbate or alleviate your pain. This will help you identify potential triggers and make necessary adjustments. For example, if you notice that certain foods increase your pain, you can avoid or limit them in your diet. If certain activities or positions worsen your pain, you can modify them or find alternative ways to accomplish the same tasks.

Next, focus on developing coping mechanisms that work for you. Chronic pain can be physically and emotionally exhausting, so it's important to have healthy ways to cope with the challenges it presents. This can include relaxation techniques like deep breathing, meditation, or guided imagery. Find activities that bring you joy and help distract from the pain, such as reading, listening to music, or engaging in hobbies. Surround yourself with a support system of friends, family, or support groups who understand your journey and can provide emotional support.

Physical activity should also be an integral part of your self-care plan. While it may seem counterintuitive to exercise when you're in pain, regular physical activity can actually help reduce pain levels and improve overall well-being. Consult with your healthcare provider or a physical therapist to identify safe and effective exercises for your specific condition. Start slowly and gradually increase the intensity and duration of your workouts. Remember to listen to your body and make adjustments as needed.

In addition to physical activity, prioritize sleep and rest. Lack of quality sleep can exacerbate pain levels and make it more difficult to cope with daily challenges. Establish a consistent sleep routine and create a sleep-friendly environment in your bedroom. Practice relaxation techniques before bed to promote better sleep quality. If you're struggling with sleep despite these efforts, consult with a healthcare professional who specializes in sleep disorders.

Lastly, remember to be kind to yourself and practice self-compassion. Living with chronic pain is not easy, and it's important to acknowledge your efforts and accomplishments. Celebrate small victories and take time to rest and recharge when needed. Set realistic expectations and be patient with yourself as you navigate the ups and downs of managing chronic pain.

Building your personalized self-care plan for chronic pain is an ongoing process. It may take time to find the right combination of strategies that work for you. Be open to trying new approaches and seeking support when needed. With perseverance and a personalized self-care plan, you can improve your quality of life and find ways to live your best life despite chronic pain.

# 7 Finding Purpose in Spite of Pain

From managing symptoms to navigating through our daily routines, it can be easy to lose sight of our passions and purpose. However, even in the midst of pain, it is possible to live a meaningful and fulfilling life. By unlocking our potential and rediscovering our passions, setting achievable goals, and overcoming isolation, we can find purpose and meaning in spite of pain. In this chapter, we will explore ways to live a purposeful life while coping with chronic pain, and how it can ultimately lead to a more fulfilling and satisfying journey.

## Rediscovering Your Passions Amidst Chronic Pain

Living with chronic pain can feel all-consuming, leaving little room for the activities and interests that used to bring us joy. It can be easy to forget what we are passionate about or to believe that we no longer have the ability to pursue those passions. However, rediscovering our passions amidst chronic pain is not only possible but can also be a powerful tool in finding purpose and meaning in our lives.

One way to start rediscovering our passions is by

reflecting on the activities or hobbies that brought us joy in the past. What were the things that made us feel alive, inspired, and fulfilled? Maybe it was painting, playing an instrument, or cooking. Whatever it may be, take the time to reconnect with those activities and see if they still bring you a sense of joy and fulfillment. If they do, consider incorporating them into your daily routine, even if it is in small doses. Rediscovering our passions can help us tap into our creativity and remind us of our unique abilities and talents.

It's important to remember that our passions don't have to be limited to physical activities. If chronic pain prevents us from engaging in activities that require physical exertion, we can explore other passions that don't rely on our bodies. It could be reading, writing, listening to music, or learning a new skill or language. The key is to find activities that spark a sense of excitement and interest within us, even if they may not be what we originally envisioned.

Rediscovering our passions amidst chronic pain also involves giving ourselves permission to adapt and modify our activities to accommodate our physical limitations. This may mean finding alternative ways to engage in our passions or seeking out support and resources that can help us adapt. For example, if we used to enjoy hiking but can no longer manage long walks, we could explore wheelchair-accessible nature trails or find virtual hiking experiences online. By adapting our passions to our current circumstances, we can still experience the joy and fulfillment they bring without worsening our pain.

Another important aspect of rediscovering our passions is being open to trying new things. Chronic pain may have forced us to let go of certain activities, but it can also open doors to new possibilities. We can use this opportunity to explore different interests and hobbies that we may have never considered before. Trying new things not only expands our horizons but also helps us discover new passions that can bring fulfillment and purpose into our lives.

In the process of rediscovering our passions amidst chronic pain, it's essential to practice self-compassion and patience. It may take time and experimentation to find activities that truly resonate with us and provide a sense of purpose. Some days may be more challenging than others, but by persistently exploring our interests and passions, we can find moments of joy and fulfillment amidst the pain.

It's also crucial to remember that rediscovering our passions is not just about finding temporary distractions from our pain. Instead, it's about nurturing our souls and reconnecting with the things that make us feel alive and whole. Our passions can act as beacons of light, guiding us through the darkness of chronic pain and reminding us of the vibrant, resilient individuals we are.

Rediscovering our passions amidst chronic pain can be a transformative journey, leading us to uncover hidden strengths, talents, and aspects of ourselves that we may have forgotten. It is a reminder that chronic pain does not define us or diminish our potential for a meaningful and fulfilling life. By embracing our passions and incorporating them into our lives, we can tap into our unique gifts and talents, finding purpose and meaning in spite of pain. So, let's take the first step towards rediscovering our passions and unlock the door to a purposeful and fulfilling life.

## Identifying your Purpose: Guiding Your Actions with a Strong Why

Living with chronic pain can make it difficult to see the purpose and meaning in our lives. It's easy to get caught up in the daily struggles of managing symptoms and navigating through our routines. However, by identifying our purpose and guiding our actions with a strong "why," we can find motivation and fulfillment even in the midst of pain.

Identifying our purpose is about understanding our deepest values, desires, and aspirations. It's about uncovering what truly matters to us and what we want to contribute to the world. When we have a clear sense of purpose, it becomes easier to align our actions with our goals and make decisions that are in line with our values.

So, how do we go about identifying our purpose amidst chronic pain? One way is through introspection and reflection. Take the time to ask yourself meaningful questions like: What do I value most in life? What brings me joy and fulfillment? What impact do I want to make in the world? These questions can help guide you towards a deeper understanding of your purpose.

Another way to identify your purpose is by examining the challenges and struggles you've faced due to chronic pain. While it's easy to view pain as a hindrance, it can also serve as a catalyst for growth and resilience. Consider the ways in which you have overcome obstacles and developed strengths through your experiences with pain. How can these experiences shape your purpose and drive you towards making a difference?

It can also be helpful to seek support and guidance from others who have gone through similar experiences. Joining support groups or connecting with individuals who understand the challenges of chronic pain can provide valuable insights and perspectives. Hearing others' stories of how they have found purpose and meaning despite their pain can inspire and motivate you on your own journey.

When identifying your purpose, it's important to keep in mind that it doesn't have to be grand or lofty. Purpose can be found in the simplest of actions and interactions. It can be as small as making someone smile or offering a listening ear to a friend in need. Remember that purpose is personal and unique to each individual.

Once you have a clearer sense of your purpose, it's crucial to use it as a guiding force in your actions. When faced with decisions or challenges, ask yourself: Does this align with my purpose? Will this contribute to my overall goals and aspirations? By continuously evaluating your actions and choices against your purpose, you can ensure that you're living a life that is meaningful and fulfilling.

In addition, having a strong "why" behind your actions can provide the motivation and perseverance needed to overcome obstacles. When pain becomes too much, reminding yourself of your purpose can give you the strength to push through and keep going. It serves as a reminder of what truly matters to you and can help you stay focused on your goals, even in the face of adversity.

Identifying your purpose and guiding your actions with a strong "why" can also help you prioritize your energy and resources. Chronic pain often requires careful management of limited energy levels, and knowing your purpose can help you determine where to direct your precious resources. By focusing on activities and pursuits that align with your purpose, you can avoid wasting energy on things that don't truly matter to you.

Ultimately, identifying your purpose and guiding your actions with a strong "why" can bring a sense of direction and meaning to your life, even in the midst of chronic pain. It's about finding what truly matters to you and aligning your actions with your values and aspirations. It's about living a life that is intentional and purposeful, despite the challenges you may face. So, take the time to reflect on your purpose, seek support from others, and let your "why" guide you towards a life of fulfillment and meaning.

## Overcoming Isolation

Living with chronic pain can be an incredibly isolating experience. It can make us feel like we are the only ones going through this struggle, causing us to withdraw from social interactions and disconnect from our support systems. The constant pain and fatigue can make it difficult to engage in activities and maintain relationships, leading to a sense of isolation and loneliness. However, it is crucial to overcome this isolation in order to live a meaningful and fulfilling life amidst chronic pain.

One way to overcome isolation is by reaching out for support. It's important to remember that you are not alone in this journey. There are many others who are going through similar experiences and can offer empathy, understanding, and guidance. Joining support groups or connecting with individuals who have firsthand experience with chronic pain can be incredibly beneficial. These groups provide a safe space to share your thoughts and feelings, receive validation, and gain valuable insights from others who truly understand what you're going through. They can also offer practical advice and coping strategies that can help you navigate the challenges of living with chronic pain.

Additionally, maintaining connections with loved ones is crucial for overcoming isolation. Chronic pain may limit your ability to engage in social activities, but that doesn't mean you have to completely withdraw from your relationships. Communicate openly with your friends and family about your limitations and needs. Let them know how they can support you and find alternative ways to spend time together. This could be as simple as having a movie night at home, playing board games, or having a video call. Even if you can't physically be present, maintaining emotional connections can go a long way in combating feelings of isolation.

It's also important to cultivate new relationships and expand your social circle. This can be done through online communities, support groups, or participating in activities that align with your interests. Finding people who share similar passions or hobbies can provide a sense of camaraderie and connection. Look for local groups or organizations that focus on activities you enjoy or would like to explore. Whether it's a book club, a knitting group, or an art class, engaging in activities with like-minded individuals can help combat isolation and create a sense of belonging.

In addition to seeking support and maintaining relationships, it's crucial to prioritize self-care. Chronic pain can be mentally and emotionally draining, so it's important to take care of your own well-being. This may involve incorporating relaxation techniques, such as deep breathing exercises or meditation, into your daily routine. It could also mean finding ways to pamper yourself, whether it's taking a warm bath, getting a massage, or indulging in a favorite hobby. Prioritizing self-care not only helps alleviate the physical and emotional toll of chronic pain but also reinforces the message that you deserve to be cared for and supported.

Overcoming isolation also involves challenging negative thoughts and beliefs. Chronic pain can often lead to feelings of worthlessness, inadequacy, or a sense of being a burden to others. It's important to recognize these thoughts and challenge them. Remind yourself that your worth is not determined by your physical abilities or limitations. You are deserving of love, support, and connection, just like anyone else. Practice self-compassion and remind yourself that chronic pain is not your fault. It's a challenge that you are facing with strength and resilience.

Engaging in meaningful activities can also help combat isolation. Find activities or pursuits that bring you joy and a sense of purpose. This could be volunteering for a cause you care about, pursuing a hobby, or engaging in creative outlets. Participating in activities that align with your passions and interests can provide a sense of fulfillment and connection to something greater than yourself. It can remind you of your unique talents and abilities and help you feel a sense of accomplishment despite the challenges of chronic pain.

Lastly, it's important to acknowledge that overcoming isolation is a process that takes time and patience. It's okay to have days where you feel more isolated or withdrawn. Be kind to yourself during these times and remind yourself that it's a normal part of the journey. Seek support from others and focus on the small steps you can take each day to combat isolation. Celebrate your progress, no matter how small, and remember that you are not defined by your pain.

Overcoming isolation is essential for living a purposeful and fulfilling life despite chronic pain. It involves seeking support, maintaining connections with loved ones, cultivating new relationships, prioritizing self-care, challenging negative thoughts, engaging in meaningful activities, and practicing patience and self-compassion. By taking these steps, you can break free from the isolation that chronic pain often brings and create a life filled with connection, purpose, and meaning. You are not alone in this journey, and together, we can overcome the challenges of chronic pain and live a life that is vibrant, fulfilling, and deeply meaningful.

# 8 Practicing Patience and Self-Compassion

It is important to remember that managing chronic pain is a journey, and like any journey, it comes with its own challenges and obstacles. In order to navigate through these fluctuations in pain, it is essential to practice patience and self-compassion. These tools can not only help individuals cope with the daily struggles of chronic pain, but also prevent and manage relapses. In this chapter, we will explore the importance of patience and self-compassion in managing chronic pain and how to incorporate them into our daily lives.

## Understanding Fluctuations in Chronic Pain

Living with chronic pain can be a rollercoaster ride, filled with unpredictable twists and turns. One day you may wake up feeling relatively pain-free, only to have a flare-up later that afternoon. It can be frustrating, disheartening, and downright exhausting. But it's important to understand that fluctuations in chronic pain are a common and normal part of the journey.

Chronic pain is often characterized by periods of increased pain intensity, known as flare-ups, followed by periods of relative relief. These fluctuations can be triggered by a variety of factors, such as physical exertion, weather changes, stress, or even something as simple as a change in daily routine. It's important to remember that these fluctuations are not a reflection of your strength or ability to cope with pain. They are simply a part of the chronic pain experience.

During a flare-up, it's natural to feel frustrated, and even defeated. You may question why this is happening to you or wonder if you'll ever experience relief. It's crucial to acknowledge and validate these feelings, but also to remind yourself that a flare-up does not mean you are failing in your journey to manage your chronic pain. It's simply a temporary setback that requires some extra attention and self-care.

One of the keys to understanding fluctuations in chronic pain is recognizing that they are not always within your control. While you can take steps to minimize the likelihood of flare-ups, such as practicing good self-care, managing stress, and following a treatment plan, it's important to accept that you cannot completely eliminate them. This can be a difficult pill to swallow, especially for individuals who are used to having control over their lives. But accepting this reality can be a freeing and empowering step towards managing chronic pain.

Understanding that fluctuations in pain are normal can also help you develop a more compassionate and patient mindset. It's easy to fall into a pattern of self-blame and negative self-talk during a flare-up. You may start to believe that you've done something wrong or that you are somehow to blame for the increased pain. But the truth is, chronic pain is a complex condition with multiple factors at play. It's not your fault, and beating yourself up will only make the situation worse.

Instead of berating yourself, practice self-compassion. Be kind and understanding towards yourself, just as you would to a close friend or loved one experiencing a difficult time. Remind yourself that pain fluctuations are a normal part of the journey, and that you are doing your best to manage them. Treat yourself with gentleness, patience, and understanding, knowing that it takes time to find the right balance and strategies to navigate through the ups and downs of chronic pain.

## Preventing and Managing Pain Relapses: Strategies to Keep You Grounded

Living with chronic pain means constantly being on guard for potential flare-ups and setbacks. While it may be impossible to completely prevent pain relapses, there are strategies you can implement to help manage them and keep yourself grounded during these challenging times.

First and foremost, it's important to prioritize self-care. This means listening to your body and giving it the rest it needs. Overexertion can often trigger flare-ups, so be mindful of your physical limits and pace yourself accordingly. Taking breaks throughout the day and practicing gentle exercises or stretches can help alleviate muscle tension and reduce the risk of pain flaring up.

Another important aspect of preventing pain relapses is stress management. Chronic pain itself can be a significant source of stress, and additional stressors can exacerbate the situation. Find healthy coping mechanisms that work for you, such as deep breathing exercises, meditation, or engaging in hobbies and activities that bring you joy. Taking time for yourself and prioritizing relaxation can help minimize the impact of stress on your pain levels.

In addition to self-care and stress management, it's crucial to stick to your treatment plan. This may include following a medication regimen, attending physical therapy sessions, or seeking alternative therapies such as acupuncture or chiropractic care. Consistency is key when it comes to managing chronic pain, and staying on top of your treatment plan can help reduce the likelihood of pain relapses.

Building a strong support system is another effective

strategy for managing pain relapses. Surround yourself with loved ones who understand and support you on your pain journey. Having people to lean on during difficult times can provide the emotional support and encouragement needed to navigate through flare-ups. Consider joining a support group where you can connect with others who are experiencing similar challenges. Sharing your experiences and learning from others can be empowering and provide valuable insights for managing pain relapses.

Additionally, it's important to communicate with your healthcare provider about your pain fluctuations. They can help you understand the underlying causes and identify potential triggers for flare-ups. Your healthcare provider may also be able to suggest additional strategies or treatment options to help prevent or manage pain relapses.

Lastly, maintaining a positive mindset and practicing mindfulness can make a significant difference in how you navigate through pain relapses. Acknowledge the challenges you face, but also focus on the progress you've made and the strategies that have helped you cope with pain in the past. Remember that pain relapses are temporary setbacks and that you have the strength and resilience to overcome them.

By implementing these strategies and being proactive in

managing pain relapses, you can keep yourself grounded and better equipped to handle the ups and downs of chronic pain. Remember that managing chronic pain is a journey, and there will be times when flare-ups occur. Be patient with yourself and continue to practice self-compassion as you navigate through these challenges. With time, you will develop a toolkit of strategies that work best for you, and the journey will become more manageable.

## The Power of Patience: Accepting the Journey

Living with chronic pain requires an immense amount of patience. It's not a journey with a clear endpoint or a quick fix. Instead, it's a path filled with twists and turns, ups and downs. Patience is a powerful tool that can help you accept the unpredictable nature of chronic pain and embrace the journey.

One of the key aspects of cultivating patience is learning to let go of the need for immediate results. It's natural to want to find a solution to your pain as quickly as possible, but the reality is that managing chronic pain takes time and experimentation. It may involve trying different treatment options, making lifestyle changes, and adapting your mindset. Be patient with yourself as you navigate through these challenges, and trust that with each step forward, you are moving closer to finding relief.

Another important aspect of patience is learning to adapt to setbacks. Chronic pain can be unpredictable, and there will be times when flare-ups occur despite your best efforts. It can be disheartening when progress feels like it's slipping away, but it's important to remember that setbacks are a natural part of the journey. Instead of viewing them as failures, see them as opportunities for growth and learning. Use setbacks as motivation to reassess your approach, seek support, and explore new strategies.

In addition to patience, acceptance is a crucial component of the journey. Acceptance doesn't mean resigning yourself to a life of pain; rather, it means acknowledging and embracing the reality of your condition. It's about accepting that chronic pain is a part of your life, but it doesn't define you. By accepting your pain, you can shift your focus from fighting against it to finding ways to work with it and live a fulfilling life despite its presence.

Practicing mindfulness can be a powerful tool in cultivating patience and acceptance. Mindfulness involves bringing your attention to the present moment and accepting it without judgment. By practicing mindfulness, you can develop a greater awareness of your pain, allowing you to respond to it with patience and self-compassion. Mindfulness can also help you detach from negative thoughts and emotions that can often arise from chronic pain, allowing you to approach your journey with a clear and focused mind.

It's important to remember that developing patience is a process. It's not something that can be achieved overnight. It requires practice and self-reflection. Be kind and gentle with yourself as you cultivate patience, and remember that it's okay to ask for help along the way. Reach out to friends, family, or support groups who can provide guidance and understanding. Surround yourself with a supportive community that can remind you to be patient.

## Building a Foundation of Self-Compassion: Steps Towards Self-kindness

Building a foundation of self-compassion is essential for anyone living with chronic pain. It involves treating yourself with kindness, understanding, and acceptance, despite the challenges you may face. Self-compassion is not always easy, especially when dealing with the ups and downs of chronic pain, but it is a skill that can be developed with practice and patience.

One of the first steps towards self-compassion is recognizing and acknowledging your pain. It can be easy to ignore or push away your pain, but doing so only prolongs the suffering. Instead, take the time to validate and honor your experience. Allow yourself to feel the emotions that arise from living with chronic pain, whether it's frustration, sadness, or anger. These emotions are valid and should not be dismissed. By acknowledging and accepting your pain, you can begin to treat yourself with the kindness and compassion you deserve.

Another important aspect of self-compassion is letting go of self-judgment. It's common for individuals with chronic pain to blame themselves or feel guilty for their condition. This self-blame is not helpful or productive. Chronic pain is a complex condition with numerous factors at play, many of which are beyond your control. It's important to remember that you are not to blame for your pain. Be gentle with yourself and release any self-judgment that may be holding you back from self-compassion.

Practicing self-care is another essential component of building self-compassion. Taking care of your physical, emotional, and mental well-being is crucial for managing chronic pain. Engage in activities that bring you joy and help you relax. Whether it's taking a warm bath, going for a walk in nature, or indulging in a hobby you love, prioritize self-care in your daily life. By dedicating time and energy to yourself, you are demonstrating self-compassion and showing yourself the love and care you deserve.

Additionally, practicing self-compassionate self-talk can have a profound impact on your well-being. Notice the negative self-talk that may arise when you experience a flare-up or setback. Instead of beating yourself up or criticizing your body, replace those negative thoughts with kind and encouraging words. Speak to yourself as you would to a close friend or loved one going through a difficult time. Remind yourself that you are doing your best, and that managing chronic pain is a challenging journey. By shifting your self-talk to be more compassionate, you can cultivate a sense of self-kindness and acceptance.

Developing a mindfulness practice can also contribute to building self-compassion. Mindfulness involves bringing your attention to the present moment without judgment. It allows you to observe your pain and emotions with curiosity and compassion. By practicing mindfulness, you can cultivate a sense of self-awareness and compassion towards your experience. You can learn to respond to pain with kindness and understanding, rather than reacting with frustration or despair.

Finally, seeking support from others can greatly enhance your self-compassion journey. Connect with friends, family, or support groups who understand and empathize with your pain. Surround yourself with individuals who can offer encouragement, understanding, and a listening ear. Sharing your experiences with others who have similar challenges can be incredibly validating and empowering. Through the support of others, you can feel less alone in your journey and continue to cultivate self-compassion.

Building a foundation of self-compassion takes time and practice. Be patient with yourself as you navigate through the ups and downs of chronic pain. Remember that self-compassion is not selfish or indulgent, but a necessary tool for managing your pain and living a fulfilling life. By treating yourself with kindness and acceptance, you can cultivate a sense of self-compassion that will guide you on your journey to managing chronic pain.

# 9 Advocating for Your Well-Being

While managing the physical and emotional toll of this condition, it can also be overwhelming to navigate the complexities of the healthcare system and ensure that your rights are being respected. However, it is important to know that there are legal options available to help you advocate for your well-being when dealing with chronic pain. In this chapter, we will discuss how you can stand up for your rights and find support through legal resources.

## Mastering the Art of Communication with Your Healthcare Providers

Living with chronic pain requires open and effective communication with your healthcare providers. This is a vital aspect of managing your condition and ensuring that you receive the care and treatment you need. In this section, we will explore some key strategies to help you master the art of communication with your healthcare providers.

First and foremost, it is essential to establish a strong foundation of trust and collaboration with your healthcare team. This begins with finding healthcare providers who specialize in chronic pain management and who genuinely listen to your concerns. Remember, you are the expert on your own pain experience, and your healthcare providers should respect and value your input.

To enhance communication with your healthcare providers, it can be helpful to come prepared for your appointments. Before your visit, make a list of any questions or concerns you have regarding your chronic pain. This will ensure that you don't forget anything important during your appointment. Additionally, consider keeping a pain journal or diary to track your symptoms, triggers, and any patterns you notice. This information can provide valuable insights to your healthcare team.

During your appointment, be proactive and assertive in expressing your needs and concerns. Clearly and concisely communicate your pain symptoms, their impact on your daily life, and any changes or new symptoms you have experienced. Don't be afraid to ask questions about your condition, treatment options, or any concerns you may have. Remember, effective communication is a two-way street, so actively listen to your healthcare provider's responses and ask for clarification if needed.

It is also crucial to communicate openly about your pain management goals and expectations. Be honest about your desired level of pain relief and how you hope to improve your quality of life. This will help your healthcare team tailor a treatment plan specifically to your needs and preferences. If a particular treatment option isn't working for you, don't hesitate to speak up and discuss alternative options. Your healthcare providers are there to support you and find the most effective solutions for managing your chronic pain.

In addition to verbal communication, non-verbal cues can also play a role in effective communication with your healthcare providers. Pay attention to your body language and facial expressions during your appointments. This can provide additional insight into your pain experience and help your healthcare team better understand your needs. Additionally, be mindful of your tone of voice and the words you choose. Communicating in a respectful and assertive manner can go a long way in fostering a positive and productive relationship with your healthcare providers.

Lastly, remember that effective communication with your healthcare providers extends beyond the walls of the clinic or hospital. Take advantage of any electronic communication tools offered by your healthcare providers, such as patient portals or email communication. These tools can help you stay connected and address any questions or concerns that may arise between appointments.

## Navigating the Complex Terrain of the Healthcare System

Navigating the healthcare system can be a daunting task, especially when dealing with chronic pain. The complex terrain of medical facilities, insurance policies, and bureaucratic processes can often feel overwhelming. However, it is essential to understand that you have the right to navigate this system with confidence and advocate for your well-being. In this section, we will explore some strategies to help you navigate the complex terrain of the healthcare system when dealing with chronic pain.

One of the first steps in navigating the healthcare system is to familiarize yourself with the resources available to you. Research and gather information about the different healthcare providers, clinics, and hospitals in your area that specialize in chronic pain management. Consider seeking recommendations from trusted sources such as your primary care physician, friends, or support groups. By doing your due diligence and choosing the right healthcare providers, you can increase your chances of receiving the care and support you need.

Once you have identified potential healthcare providers, it is crucial to understand your insurance coverage and any limitations or requirements that may be in place. Familiarize yourself with your insurance policy, including what services are covered, any required pre-authorizations, and potential out-of-pocket expenses. Understanding your insurance coverage will help you navigate the financial aspect of your healthcare and ensure that you can access the treatments and medications you need without undue financial burden.

Another aspect of navigating the healthcare system is coordinating your care among multiple providers. Chronic pain often requires a multidisciplinary approach, involving specialists such as pain management physicians, physical therapists, psychologists, and others. It is important to ensure that these providers communicate and coordinate your care effectively. Keep a record of your healthcare team's contact information and make sure they have access to your medical records, test results, and treatment plans. This will help facilitate effective collaboration and prevent any gaps in your care.

As you navigate the healthcare system, it is essential to be an active participant in your own healthcare. Be proactive in asking questions, seeking clarification, and understanding your treatment options. Research and educate yourself about your condition, potential treatments, and alternative therapies. This knowledge will empower you to make informed decisions and advocate for the treatments and interventions that are best suited for your needs.

In addition to advocating for yourself, it can be beneficial to seek support from patient advocacy organizations or support groups. These groups can provide valuable resources, information, and emotional support. They can also help you navigate the healthcare system by providing guidance, connecting you with experienced individuals who have faced similar challenges, and advocating for systemic changes to improve the care and treatment of chronic pain patients.

Lastly, don't hesitate to assert your rights as a patient. If you encounter any barriers or face discrimination within the healthcare system, know that you have the right to speak up and take action. This can include filing complaints with the appropriate regulatory bodies, seeking legal counsel, or reaching out to patient advocacy organizations for guidance.

Navigating the complex terrain of the healthcare system when dealing with chronic pain may not be easy, but by educating yourself, seeking support, and being proactive, you can effectively advocate for your well-being. Remember that you are not alone in this journey, and there are resources available to help you overcome the challenges you may face. Together, we can work towards a healthcare system that respects and supports the rights and needs of chronic pain patients.

## Understanding Your Legal Rights as a Chronic Pain Patient

Living with chronic pain not only takes a toll on your physical and emotional well-being, but it can also present unique legal challenges. As a chronic pain patient, it is essential to understand your legal rights and the resources available to you to advocate for your well-being. In this section, we will explore the legal aspects of dealing with chronic pain and provide you with valuable information to help you navigate this complex terrain.

One of the fundamental legal rights you have as a chronic pain patient is the right to access appropriate medical care and treatment. This means that healthcare providers are obligated to provide you with the necessary care to manage your pain effectively. If you feel that your healthcare provider is not adequately addressing your pain or is denying you access to necessary treatments, it may be necessary to assert your rights and seek legal advice.

In addition to the right to appropriate medical care, chronic pain patients also have the right to be treated with respect, dignity, and compassion. You should not be subjected to discrimination or stigma due to your pain condition. If you experience any form of mistreatment or discrimination, it is essential to understand that you have legal recourse. Document any instances of discrimination or mistreatment, and consult with a legal professional to discuss your options.

Another crucial legal right for chronic pain patients is the right to access your medical records. Having access to your medical records is important for several reasons. It allows you to stay informed about your treatment, understand your condition, and actively participate in decisions about your care. If you encounter any obstacles or resistance when trying to access your medical records, it is important to understand that you have legal rights in this area as well.

Chronic pain patients also have the right to informed consent. Informed consent means that healthcare providers must provide you with all the information necessary to make an informed decision about your treatment. This includes information about the potential risks, benefits, and alternatives to a particular treatment. If you feel that you have not been adequately informed about your treatment options, you have the right to seek additional information and ask questions to make an informed decision about your care.

It is crucial to understand that navigating the legal aspects of chronic pain can be challenging. Laws and regulations vary depending on your jurisdiction, and the healthcare system itself can be complex. That is why it is essential to seek legal advice from professionals who specialize in healthcare and disability law. They can provide you with the guidance and support you need to navigate the legal system and advocate for your rights effectively.

In addition to legal professionals, there are also resources available that can help you understand your rights and provide you with support. Patient advocacy organizations, support groups, and online communities can provide valuable information and connect you with individuals who have faced similar legal challenges. These resources can offer guidance, share experiences, and help you navigate the legal aspects of chronic pain.

## Moving Forward: Effective Self-Advocacy Strategies

In this section, we will discuss some effective self-advocacy strategies that can help you navigate the challenges of living with chronic pain and ensure that your needs are met.

First and foremost, it's crucial to educate yourself about

your condition and the available treatment options. Knowledge is power, and the more you understand about your chronic pain, the better equipped you will be to communicate with healthcare providers and make informed decisions about your care. Research different treatment modalities, alternative therapies, and lifestyle changes that may help alleviate your pain. This information will not only empower you but also give you confidence when discussing your treatment options with healthcare providers.

Next, build a support network of individuals who understand and empathize with your pain experience. Connecting with others who are going through similar struggles can provide a sense of validation, encouragement, and valuable insights. Joining support groups, both in-person and online, can help you share experiences, exchange coping strategies, and find emotional support. Additionally, patient advocacy organizations can offer resources, guidance, and a platform to voice your concerns and advocate for systemic changes in the healthcare system.

Effective self-advocacy also involves setting clear goals for your pain management and overall well-being. Take the time to reflect on what you hope to achieve through your treatment and what improvements you want to see in your quality of life. By clearly defining your goals, you can better communicate them to your healthcare team and work together to create a tailored treatment plan. Remember, you are an active participant in your care, and your input is essential for finding the most effective solutions for managing your chronic pain.

In addition to setting goals, it's important to establish open lines of communication with your healthcare providers. Keep a journal to track your symptoms, triggers, and any patterns you notice. Share this information with your healthcare team to provide them with a comprehensive understanding of your pain experience. Be open and honest about your concerns, questions, and treatment preferences. Effective communication involves not only speaking up but also actively listening to your healthcare providers' expertise and recommendations. Ask for clarification when needed and collaborate with your healthcare team to find the best strategies for managing your pain.

When facing barriers or challenges within the healthcare system, it's essential to remain persistent and assertive in advocating for your rights. If you feel that your pain is not being adequately addressed, explore other treatment options or seek a second opinion. Don't be afraid to speak up if you encounter discrimination or mistreatment. Document any instances of mistreatment and consult with a legal professional if necessary. Remember that you have the right to be treated with respect, dignity, and compassion, and don't hesitate to assert those rights when needed.

Finally, take care of your overall well-being. Chronic pain can be emotionally and mentally draining, so it's important to prioritize self-care and seek out activities that bring you joy and relaxation. This could include practicing mindfulness or meditation, engaging in gentle exercise or movement, or pursuing hobbies and interests that distract from your pain. Taking care of your mental and emotional well-being is just as important as managing your physical pain.

In conclusion, effective self-advocacy is crucial for managing chronic pain and ensuring that your needs are met within the healthcare system. By educating yourself, building a support network, setting clear goals, communicating openly with your healthcare providers, and assertively advocating for your rights, you can navigate the challenges of chronic pain with confidence. Remember that you are not alone, and there are resources available to support you on your journey towards better pain management and overall well-being.

# 10 Thriving Beyond Pain to Create a Brighter Future

From daily activities to long-term goals, the pain can feel like a tremendously overwhelming obstacle. However, despite the difficulties, it is possible to not only survive but thrive with chronic pain. In fact, many individuals have experienced a phenomenon known as Post-Traumatic Growth, where they have found a renewed sense of purpose and resilience in the face of chronic pain. In this chapter, we will explore how you can create a brighter future and live fully with chronic pain through the power of Post-Traumatic Growth.

## Understanding Post-Traumatic Growth in Chronic Pain Patients

Living with chronic pain is a complex and challenging experience that can take a toll on every aspect of a person's life. The pain can be debilitating, affecting daily activities, relationships, and even long-term goals and dreams.

However, amidst the darkness, there is a glimmer of hope. Many individuals living with chronic pain have experienced a phenomenon known as Post-Traumatic Growth. This concept refers to the positive psychological changes that can occur after a traumatic event, such as living with chronic pain. It is the idea that despite the pain and suffering, individuals can find a renewed sense of purpose, strength, and resilience.

Post-Traumatic Growth is not about denying the difficulties or minimizing the pain. It is about acknowledging the challenges and embracing the potential for personal growth and transformation. It's about shifting our perspective and finding new meaning in our lives, despite the chronic pain.

One of the key elements of Post-Traumatic Growth is the recognition that pain and suffering can be transformative. It forces us to confront our limitations, reevaluate our priorities, and tap into our inner strength. It can be a catalyst for personal growth, leading us to develop new coping mechanisms, deepen our relationships, and find a sense of purpose and meaning in our lives.

Research has shown that individuals who experience Post-Traumatic Growth often report positive changes in several areas of their lives. These changes can include a greater appreciation for life, improved relationships, increased personal strength, spiritual growth, and a new perspective on their values and priorities. While everyone's journey is unique, these changes are often characterized by a deeper understanding of oneself, increased resilience, and a greater sense of gratitude for the present moment.

The process of experiencing Post-Traumatic Growth is not linear, and it can take time. It's important to give yourself permission to grieve, to feel the pain, and to process the emotions that come with living with chronic pain. It's not about pretending that everything is fine; it's about embracing the pain and using it as a catalyst for growth and transformation.

One of the first steps towards embracing Post-Traumatic Growth is shifting our mindset from a victim mentality to one of empowerment. It's about acknowledging that while we may not have control over our pain, we have control over how we respond to it. This shift in perspective can open the door to new possibilities and a brighter future.

Another important aspect of Post-Traumatic Growth is seeking support from others who have experienced similar challenges. Connecting with a support group, joining an online community, or finding a therapist who specializes in chronic pain can be incredibly beneficial. These individuals can offer understanding, empathy, and guidance as we navigate the complexities of living with chronic pain. They can also provide practical tips and strategies for managing pain and improving our overall well-being.

Additionally, practicing self-care is essential in the journey towards Post-Traumatic Growth. Taking care of our physical, emotional, and mental health is crucial for developing resilience and finding joy in the midst of chronic pain. This can include activities such as gentle exercise, meditation, journaling, engaging in hobbies, and spending time with loved ones. Finding what brings us joy and incorporating it into our daily lives can have a profound impact on our overall well-being.

It's important to remember that experiencing Post-Traumatic Growth does not mean that the pain goes away or that life becomes perfect. Living with chronic pain will always present challenges, and there will be difficult days. However, by embracing the concept of Post-Traumatic Growth, we can cultivate a mindset of resilience and positivity, even in the face of adversity.

## Paving the Way for a Positive Future with Chronic Pain

Living with chronic pain can be incredibly challenging, but it doesn't mean that you can't have a positive future. In fact, by embracing the concept of Post-Traumatic Growth, you can pave the way for a brighter future despite the pain.

One important aspect of paving the way for a positive

future is to cultivate resilience. Resilience is the ability to bounce back from difficult experiences and adapt to change. It's about developing the mental and emotional strength to overcome challenges and find meaning and purpose in your life. While chronic pain may make it harder to bounce back, it is still possible with the right mindset and support.

To cultivate resilience, it's essential to focus on self-care. Taking care of yourself physically, mentally, and emotionally is crucial for building resilience and finding joy in the midst of chronic pain. This can include gentle exercise, such as stretching or walking, to keep your body moving and improve circulation. It can also involve practicing relaxation techniques, such as deep breathing or meditation, to reduce stress and promote a sense of calm. Additionally, engaging in activities that bring you joy and fulfillment, such as hobbies or spending time with loved ones, can boost your overall well-being and resilience.

Another important aspect of paving the way for a positive future is to reframe your perspective. Instead of seeing chronic pain as a barrier, try to view it as an opportunity for growth and transformation. Pain can be a powerful teacher, forcing us to slow down, reassess our priorities, and find new ways of approaching life. By reframing your perspective, you can find meaning and purpose even in the midst of pain.

It's also important to surround yourself with a supportive community. Connecting with others who have experienced similar challenges can provide empathy, understanding, and guidance. Support groups, online communities, or therapy sessions specifically tailored for individuals with chronic pain can be invaluable sources of support. These individuals can offer practical tips and strategies for managing pain, as well as emotional support to help you navigate the ups and downs of living with chronic pain.

In addition to building resilience and finding support, it's important to set realistic goals and expectations. Living with chronic pain may require you to make adjustments and accommodations in various aspects of your life. Setting achievable goals and adapting to your limitations can help you maintain a sense of control and accomplishment. Remember that it's okay to modify your goals or adjust your expectations as needed. It's about finding a balance between pushing yourself and taking care of yourself.

Finding purpose and meaning in your life can also pave the way for a positive future with chronic pain. Despite the limitations and challenges, there are still ways to make a meaningful impact in the world. This can involve pursuing hobbies or interests that bring you joy, volunteering for causes that resonate with you, or finding ways to share your story and help others going through similar experiences. By finding purpose and meaning, you can create a sense of fulfillment and a positive outlook on the future.

Lastly, practicing gratitude can be a powerful tool for paving the way to a positive future. Chronic pain can easily consume your thoughts and emotions, making it difficult to see beyond the pain. However, by focusing on what you are grateful for, you can shift your mindset and find joy in the present moment. Take time each day to reflect on the things you are grateful for, whether it's the support of loved ones, moments of pain relief, or small victories and accomplishments. Cultivating gratitude can bring a sense of peace and optimism, even in the midst of chronic pain.

Living fully with chronic pain is not easy, but it is possible. By embracing the concept of Post-Traumatic Growth and adopting strategies to build resilience, find support, set realistic goals, and find purpose and meaning, you can pave the way for a positive future. Remember that each journey is unique, and it's okay to have difficult days. Allow yourself to feel the pain, but also embrace the potential for growth and transformation. With the right mindset and support, you can thrive and live fully, even with chronic pain.

# Appendix

## Recommended Reads: Self-Help Books for Chronic Pain Management

There are numerous self-help books available that can provide valuable insights, tips, and strategies for managing chronic pain and improving your quality of life. In this section, we will explore some recommended reads that can empower you to take control of your pain and live a more fulfilling life.

1. "Managing Chronic Pain: A Cognitive-Behavioral Therapy Approach" by John Otis

Cognitive-Behavioral Therapy (CBT) has been proven to be effective in managing chronic pain. This book, written by a renowned pain management specialist, provides a comprehensive guide to understanding and applying CBT techniques for pain relief. It offers practical exercises and strategies to help you identify and change negative thoughts and behaviors that may contribute to your pain experience. With this book, you will learn how to develop healthy coping mechanisms and improve your overall well-being.

2. "The Pain Survival Guide: How to Reclaim Your Life" by Dennis Turk and Frits Winter

Dennis Turk and Frits Winter, both experts in pain

management, offer practical advice and strategies in their book "The Pain Survival Guide." This comprehensive guide covers a range of topics, including understanding pain, medication management, relaxation techniques, and maintaining an active lifestyle. It also provides valuable insights into the emotional impact of chronic pain and offers strategies for coping with depression, anxiety, and stress. With its holistic approach, this book will empower you to take control of your pain and live a fulfilling life.

3. "You Are Not Your Pain: Using Mindfulness to Relieve Pain, Reduce Stress, and Restore Well-Being" by Vidyamala Burch and Danny Penman

Mindfulness has gained significant recognition as an effective tool for managing chronic pain. In "You Are Not Your Pain," Vidyamala Burch and Danny Penman offer a practical and accessible guide to using mindfulness techniques to alleviate pain and improve well-being. This book provides step-by-step instructions for various mindfulness practices, such as meditation and body scanning, as well as strategies for incorporating mindfulness into everyday life. By learning to be present with your pain, you can cultivate a sense of peace and acceptance.

4. "Living Well with Pain and Illness: The Mindful Way to Free Yourself from Suffering" by Vidyamala

Burch

Vidyamala Burch, a mindfulness teacher and pain management expert, shares her personal journey with chronic pain in "Living Well with Pain and Illness." This book combines personal anecdotes, practical advice, and mindfulness techniques to guide readers towards a more compassionate and fulfilling life despite the challenges of chronic pain. Burch emphasizes the importance of self-compassion, acceptance, and mindfulness in managing pain and offers exercises and meditations to cultivate these qualities.

5. "The Chronic Pain Care Workbook: A Self-Treatment Approach to Pain Relief" by Michael J. Lewandowski

"The Chronic Pain Care Workbook" provides a comprehensive and self-guided approach to managing chronic pain. Michael J. Lewandowski, a licensed psychologist, combines cognitive-behavioral therapy, acceptance and commitment therapy, and mindfulness techniques in this practical workbook. It offers step-by-step exercises, worksheets, and tools to help you develop coping strategies, improve communication with healthcare providers, and create an individualized pain management plan. With this workbook, you can actively participate in your own healing process and find relief from chronic pain.

These are just a few of the many self-help books available for managing chronic pain. Each book offers unique insights and strategies, so it may be beneficial to explore multiple resources to find the approaches that resonate with you. Remember, managing chronic pain is a personal journey, and what works for one person may not work for another. It's important to find the resources and techniques that align with your values and needs.

In addition to self-help books, it may also be helpful to seek out support groups and networks specifically designed for individuals living with chronic pain. These communities can provide a safe and understanding space for sharing experiences, gaining support, and learning from others who are on a similar journey. The next section will explore the power of community and the benefits of online support groups and networks for individuals with chronic pain.

As you embark on your journey towards managing chronic pain, remember that you are not alone. There is a wealth of resources and support available to help you along the way. By investing time in educating yourself and exploring different strategies, you can empower yourself to reclaim your life and live well despite chronic pain. Never surrender to your pain; take the first step today towards a better quality of life.

## The Power of Community: Online Support Groups and Networks

Living with chronic pain can often make you feel isolated and alone. The constant battle with pain can take a toll on your mental and emotional well-being. That's why finding a community of people who understand what you're going through can be incredibly powerful and healing. Online support groups and networks provide a safe space for individuals with chronic pain to connect, share experiences, and learn from one another. In this section, we will explore the power of community and the benefits of online support groups and networks for individuals living with chronic pain.

One of the key benefits of online support groups is the opportunity to connect with others who are going through similar experiences. Chronic pain can be a complex and often invisible condition, making it difficult for others to fully understand what you're going through. Being a part of a community that understands your struggles can provide a sense of validation and relief. It allows you to connect with people who truly understand your challenges, frustrations, and triumphs.

In online support groups, you can share your

experiences, ask questions, and receive support from individuals who have been in similar situations. These groups often serve as a platform for members to exchange advice, tips, and coping strategies. It can be incredibly empowering to hear firsthand from others who have found ways to manage their pain and improve their quality of life. By sharing your own experiences, you can also help others who may be going through similar struggles, creating a sense of camaraderie and support.

Online support groups also provide a space for emotional support and validation. Living with chronic pain can bring about a range of emotions, including frustration, anger, sadness, and anxiety. It can be incredibly beneficial to have a community where you can freely express these emotions without judgment. In online support groups, you can find comfort in knowing that you are not alone in your emotional journey. Others can offer advice, encouragement, and empathy, reminding you that your feelings are valid and understandable.

Another advantage of online support groups is the convenience and accessibility they offer. Living with chronic pain often comes with physical limitations, making it difficult to attend in-person support groups or events. Online support groups eliminate these barriers by providing a platform for connection from the comfort of your own home. This accessibility allows individuals from all walks of life, regardless of their location or physical abilities, to participate and benefit from the support and resources available.

In addition to the emotional support and practical advice, online support groups can also serve as a valuable source of information. Members often share resources, articles, and recommendations for managing chronic pain. This collective knowledge can help you stay informed about the latest treatments, therapies, and research in the field of pain management. It's important to note that while online support groups can provide valuable information, it's always essential to consult with a healthcare professional before implementing any new strategies or treatments.

When seeking out online support groups and networks, it's important to find communities that align with your values and needs. Some groups may focus on specific conditions or treatments, while others may have a broader focus on chronic pain in general. Take the time to research and explore different groups to find ones that resonate with you. Consider factors such as the group's size, rules and guidelines, and the level of activity and engagement.

Social media platforms such as Facebook and Reddit often have dedicated groups and communities focused on chronic pain. These platforms allow for easy connection and interaction with other members. There are also websites and forums specifically designed for individuals living with chronic pain, offering a more structured and moderated environment. Exploring these platforms can help you find the community that best suits your needs.

In addition to online support groups, there are also virtual events and webinars that provide opportunities for education and connection. Many organizations and healthcare providers offer online workshops, conferences, and seminars on various topics related to chronic pain. Attending these virtual events can not only expand your knowledge but also provide opportunities to connect with experts and fellow individuals living with chronic pain.

It's important to remember that while online support groups and networks can be incredibly valuable, they are not a substitute for professional medical advice. It's always essential to consult with a healthcare professional for personalized guidance and treatment options. However, these communities can complement and enhance your overall pain management plan by providing support, information, and a sense of belonging.

## Chronically Happy: A Pain and Symptom Tracking Journal

It can be difficult to keep track of all the different symptoms and triggers that come with this condition. That's where a pain and symptom tracking journal comes in. This tool allows you to record and monitor your pain levels, symptoms, and any patterns or triggers that may be causing them. Not only can it help you better understand your condition, but it can also provide valuable information to your healthcare team. In this section, we'll explore the benefits of using a pain and symptom tracking journal and how it can help you find moments of happiness amidst the challenges of living with chronic pain.

One powerful tool that can make a significant difference in this journey is a pain and symptom tracking journal.

Tracking your symptoms may not be the first thing that comes to mind when dealing with chronic pain, but it is an essential aspect of managing and understanding your condition. Here's why:

1. Gaining Insight and Awareness: Tracking your symptoms allows you to gain a deeper understanding of your condition. It helps you identify patterns, triggers,

and potential causes of your pain and discomfort. By consistently recording your symptoms, you can start to see connections between certain activities, foods, weather conditions, or emotional states and the severity or frequency of your symptoms. This awareness is crucial in developing effective coping strategies and making informed decisions about your health.

2. Enhancing Communication with Healthcare Professionals: When you visit your healthcare team, being able to provide detailed information about your symptoms and their patterns can greatly enhance the effectiveness of your appointments. A pain and symptom tracking journal provides a clear record of your experiences, enabling you to communicate your concerns and challenges more accurately. This can help your healthcare professionals tailor their treatment plans, adjust medications, or explore new approaches to managing your pain.

3. Facilitating Collaboration and Empowerment: With a pain and symptom tracking journal, you become an active participant in your own healthcare. It empowers you to take control of your condition by providing you with valuable information to share with your healthcare team. This collaborative approach encourages open discussions, enables you to ask informed questions, and ensures that your treatment plan aligns with your specific needs and goals.

4. Identifying Triggers and Solutions: Tracking your symptoms can help you identify triggers that worsen your pain or discomfort. Whether it's certain activities, foods, environmental factors, or emotional stressors, identifying these triggers allows you to make necessary changes in your lifestyle and daily routine. By avoiding or minimizing these triggers, you can potentially reduce the severity or frequency of your symptoms and improve your overall well-being.

5. Celebrating Progress and Success: Chronic pain management is a journey, and sometimes it can be challenging to see the progress you're making. A pain and symptom tracking journal provides a tangible record of your experiences and allows you to celebrate even the smallest victories. You can look back and see how far you've come, acknowledge the positive changes you've made, and find moments of happiness and resilience amidst the challenges.

***Transforming Data into Action: Analyzing Your Tracker's Insights***

Now that you've been diligently tracking your pain levels, symptoms, and triggers in your pain and symptom tracking journal, it's time to dive into the valuable insights that your tracker can provide. Tracking your symptoms is not just about documenting your experiences; it's about transforming that data into actionable information that can guide your treatment and improve your overall well-being.

When it comes to analyzing your tracker's insights, there are a few key steps you can take to make the most out of the data you've collected. Let's explore these steps in more detail:

1. Review your tracker regularly: The first step in analyzing your tracker's insights is to review it regularly. Set aside dedicated time to go through your entries and look for patterns or trends. By doing this consistently, you can spot any changes or correlations between your symptoms and potential triggers.

2. Look for correlations and patterns: As you review your tracker, pay close attention to any correlations or patterns that emerge. Are there certain activities, foods, or environmental factors that consistently coincide with increased pain or discomfort? Are there any times of day or weather conditions that seem to have an impact on your symptoms? Identifying these patterns can help you pinpoint potential triggers and make necessary adjustments to your daily routine or lifestyle.

3. Consider the context: When analyzing your tracker's insights, it's important to consider the context surrounding your symptoms. Take note of any

significant events, stressors, or changes in your life that may have influenced your symptoms. Understanding the broader context can provide valuable information and help you make connections between your physical well-being and your emotional state or external factors.

4. Consult with your healthcare team: Your pain and symptom tracking journal is not meant to replace the expertise of your healthcare team. Once you've analyzed your tracker's insights, it's essential to consult with your healthcare professionals. Share your findings, discuss any patterns or correlations you've identified, and ask for their input and guidance. They can provide valuable insights, offer additional perspectives, and help you make informed decisions about your treatment plan.

5. Adjust your treatment plan: Armed with the insights from your pain and symptom tracking journal and the guidance of your healthcare team, it may be necessary to make adjustments to your treatment plan. This could involve changes in medication dosage or frequency, modifications to your lifestyle or daily routine, or the addition of new approaches to managing your pain. Your tracker's insights can serve as a roadmap for optimizing your treatment and improving your quality of life.

6. Monitor progress and adapt: As you implement

changes to your treatment plan, continue to monitor your progress and adapt as needed. Keep tracking your symptoms to see how the adjustments you've made are affecting your well-being. Celebrate the positive changes and resilience you've shown along the way, and be open to making further modifications if necessary. Remember, managing chronic pain is an ongoing process, and your pain and symptom tracking journal is a tool that can help you navigate that journey.

By analyzing your tracker's insights and using them as a guide for your treatment, you can make informed decisions, better manage your pain, and improve your overall well-being.

*Encouraging Stories: Successes of Using a Symptom Tracker*

It's easy to lose hope and become discouraged by the constant discomfort and limitations it brings. However, by using a pain and symptom tracking journal, many individuals have found renewed hope and empowerment in managing their condition. Here are some inspiring stories of success from individuals who have used a symptom tracker to take control of their chronic pain journey.

Mary, a 45-year-old woman who has been living with fibromyalgia for over a decade, found that keeping a pain and symptom tracking journal was a game-changer in her pain management. Before using a tracker, she struggled to identify what triggered her flare-ups and couldn't effectively communicate her symptoms to her healthcare team. However, once she started recording her pain levels, daily activities, and potential triggers, patterns began to emerge. Mary discovered that certain foods, particularly processed sugars, were exacerbating her pain. Armed with this newfound knowledge, she made dietary changes and noticed a significant reduction in the frequency and severity of her flare-ups. Mary's symptom tracker gave her the power to make informed decisions about her health and take proactive steps towards improving her well-being.

John, a 32-year-old man living with chronic back pain, used his pain and symptom tracking journal to identify how his emotions impacted his pain levels. Through consistent tracking, he realized that his pain tended to intensify during periods of high stress or anxiety. With this knowledge, John was able to incorporate stress management techniques such as meditation and relaxation exercises into his daily routine. Over time, he noticed a significant decrease in his pain levels and an overall improvement in his emotional well-being. John's story highlights the power of tracking not only physical symptoms but also emotional states, as they can greatly impact pain levels and overall quality of life.

Another success story comes from Sarah, a 55-year-old woman living with rheumatoid arthritis. Before using a pain and symptom tracking journal, Sarah felt frustrated by the unpredictability of her symptoms. She couldn't identify any specific triggers and felt helpless in managing her pain. However, once she started diligently recording her pain levels, joint stiffness, and daily activities, she noticed a pattern. Sarah realized that certain weather conditions, particularly cold and damp days, were consistently associated with increased pain and stiffness. Armed with this information, she was able to plan her activities and adjust her self-care routines accordingly. By avoiding unnecessary exposure to cold and dampness, Sarah experienced a significant reduction in pain and improved her overall quality of life.

These inspiring stories highlight the value of using a pain and symptom tracking journal in managing chronic pain. By tracking and analyzing their symptoms, individuals like Mary, John, and Sarah were able to gain insight into their conditions, communicate effectively with their healthcare teams, identify triggers, and make necessary changes to their lifestyles. Their journeys show us that while chronic pain may present daily challenges, it doesn't have to define our lives.

By adopting a proactive and empowered approach to pain management, you too can find moments of happiness amidst the challenges. Whether it's through a pain and symptom tracking journal like Chronically Happy or another method that works for you, the key is to take control of your own healthcare journey.

www.ingramcontent.com/pod-product-compliance
Lightning Source LLC
Chambersburg PA
CBHW050918260726
48660CB00001B/277